Superstar Fitness

GRAEME HILDITCH

Superstar
Fitness

DISCOVER THE TRAINING SECRETS OF
WORLD'S BEST FOOTBALLERS

JOHN BLAKE

Published by John Blake Publishing Ltd,
3 Bramber Court, 2 Bramber Road,
London W14 9PB, England

www.johnblakepublishing.co.uk

First published in paperback in 2010

ISBN: 978-1-84454-695-4

British Library Cataloguing-in-Publication Data:

A catalogue record for this book is available from the British Library.

Design by www.envydesign.co.uk

Printed in Great Britain by CPI Bookmarque Ltd, Croydon, CR0 4TD

1 3 5 7 9 10 8 6 4 2

Papers used by John Blake Publishing are natural, recyclable products made
from wood grown in sustainable forests. The manufacturing processes conform
to the environmental regulations of the country of origin.

While every effort has been made to ensure the accuracy and reliability
of the information contained within this book, the author and publisher cannot
take responsibility for any injury sustained whatsoever as a result of engaging
with any of the activities described in the text. All instructions are intended
purely as general guidelines and should not under any circumstances be
used in the place of qualified medical advice. Always consult a doctor
before engaging in exercise.

The Multistage Fitness Test, also known as the bleep test, is now established
as the most reliable and easy-to-use fitness test. It is used in talent
identification programmes across the globe, in schools and clubs and by
the emergency services and armed forces to determine fitness levels.
To purchase this resource contact Coachwise 1st4sport. 0113 201 5555,
Chelsea Close, Amberley Road, Leeds LS12 4UP. www.1st4sport.com

CONTENTS

INTRODUCTION

The World Cup, FA Cup Final, Champions League Final and the game which will clinch the Premiership title: the build-up to a major football final always gets the press worked up into a frenzy of excitement. In the days running up to the climax of a tournament, any past feud between players or managers is dug up and the salivating media circus stirs and asks the big questions everyone wants answered.

Who's going to win and by how much? Who's going to score? Who will lose the plot and start throwing punches? Will Ronaldo be booked for time wasting for reshaping his hair? Will Beckham get through a match without someone in the crowd insulting his wife?

The media attention surrounding big games is nothing out of the ordinary and very much expected by players and supporters alike but one subject is rarely explored at any time of the season, let alone before two of the best teams in Europe or the world lock horns. How do the players condition their bodies to meet the demands of the modern game?

What is involved in conditioning the legs of the Premiership stars who spend nine or even ten months of the year playing the beautiful game? The press may gloss over it, but we want to know if there is any way us mere mortals can replicate their training secrets to give us a few extra few yards of pace or that extra energy boost in the dying minutes of a Sunday league match.

Win or lose, when the final whistle blows at the end of a big cup final, players of the top teams such as Manchester United, Liverpool, Chelsea and Arsenal will have played well over 60-70 games of football since the beginning of the season – and that's not including reporting for international duty.

With more money than ever being poured into the game, so the number of matches per season is bumped up to give the viewing public the entertainment and value that their gate ticket or Sky subscription deserves. Players for these top teams who have dominated the game for the best part of a decade will be expected to play a staggering amount of football in a season with very little time between games to recover from health niggles.

At the close of the modern season, the statistics of matches played and the hours of playing time is mind blowing:

Premiership	38 games
FA Cup	14 games
Carling Cup	7 games
Champions League	16 games
Internationals	10 games
Total	**85 games**

Of course, not all teams will reach the finals of the major tournaments every year – but suppose they did? Without extra time, that's a staggering 127 hours (7650 minutes) of football from August until May, averaging out at an average of 212 minutes a week. These figures are approximate but it gives you a rough idea of how much running the top players will have to do week in week out to be the best in the world.

Whatever your opinion of their much-publicised playboy antics – both on and off the pitch – just the fact that the elite players manage to maintain this level and intensity of exercise over the course of a season is incredible.

So how do they do it and what tips can recreational footballers use to help them improve their fitness and improve their game?

As a personal trainer who works closely with competitive athletes, I naturally have a good idea of what is involved in sports-specific conditioning and the various modalities of training required to meet the demands of the game, but until now I have never actually known for sure the precise fitness regimes of top class footballers.

So, with the help of some of the fitness and strength coaches from the Premiership's biggest clubs, I have managed to find out some of the tips and tricks that their footballers use to keep off the physio's bench and out on the pitch playing the game.

Thanks to the cooperation of the players themselves, their fitness coaches and my own background in sports nutrition and injury prevention/treatment, I have managed to compile priceless information that any footballer of any ability can relate to and hopefully use to their full advantage to give their game that extra edge.

Throughout the book, you will discover fascinating facts about precision fitness training which you can use in your pre-season preparations, no matter what your level of ability. Whether you play competitively at school or knock lumps out of your mates in a five-a-side match once a week you will learn just how small changes to a nutritional programme or training session can enhance performance – or, if done incorrectly, diminish it.

For example, did you know that by performing a highly specific type of hamstring stretch, you can significantly increase blood flow to the legs? By comparison, other commonly-used stretches often leave the leg muscles sleepy and unresponsive. By performing highly specific stretches, you can warm your legs up far more effectively, waking up the whole nervous system and making the difference between your legs feeling lazy before stretching to them bursting with energy and ready to run circles round the opposition.

Then there are dozens of little nutrition secrets which the stars use to give them that edge. Did you know that ingesting a certain amount of caffeine before a game can increase your anaerobic capacity and make you perform harder for longer?

This book has been written to give you an insight into the fitness lives of the game's top players and also provide a number of invaluable tips used by the likes of Ronaldo and Lampard, which you can incorporate into your own football training and improve your game.

You may not have access to your choice of physiotherapist, physiologist, massage therapist or sports nutritionist but by following the information in this book you will have the next best thing.

CHAPTER ONE

MAKE-UP OF A PREMIERSHIP FOOTBALLER

Although I'm not the greatest fan of the sometimes puerile attitudes demonstrated towards officials or the award-winning theatricals which are performed in the box by certain Premiership players, I do have a huge amount of respect for their physicality and how they do what they do at such a pace and intensity.

This chapter looks at the make-up (not the cosmetic type) of elite football players and what physiological attributes makes their bodies the ideal football playing machine and, more importantly, what you can do to get yourself into the best physical shape you can with your own genes. Irrespective of player ability, everyone has their own top level of fitness which they can aspire to. Although it can safely be said that the Premiership's elite are all genetically gifted and possess innately superior levels of fitness to the likes of you and I, many of them still have to work hard at their fitness to achieve the physical demands of the game over the course of a season.

Over the years, first class football has seen interesting characters tear around the pitch, with a select few attracting pretty harsh attention from the media for less-than-athletic physiques. Players such as the legendary Wales and Everton keeper Neville Southall and Liverpool's Neil Ruddock copped a lot of stick over the years for being chief suspects in the case of who-ate-all-the-pies. But amazingly, despite sporting what you'd describe as less than athletic physiques, match-winning performances from both players, particularly Southall, have made them heroic figures in the game to this day. However, these days, very few of the Premiership players can get away with non-standard fitness levels and physiques.

Since its inception in 1992, the Premiership has been worth an incredible amount of money and even though many of its top clubs are around a whopping £300m in the red, they continue to pump money into the league and pay crazy money for the world's best players. The result is that clubs expect their players to deliver and with their price tag comes a huge amount of pressure to win every game and get the silverware. If players do not meet the minimum requirements that the club sets them in terms of physical fitness and performance, they might as well forget their £80,000 a week jobs and live life like the rest of us mortals.

This point was perfectly illustrated by World Cup-winning legend Argentinean Ossie Ardiles. Even Ardiles, arguably the best player of his generation, admitted just after he retired in 1991 that big changes started to happen in terms of optimising the physical performance of every player. They may have been gifted, but that gift had to be honed and taken to its peak, essentially so that the clubs could reap the (financial as well as silverware) rewards.

In an article in *The Times* Ardiles compared the attitudes towards fitness in his glory days during the '70s with those to be heard in 2009. 'Now it is completely different,' he revealed. 'Players have learnt to look after their body and managers have learnt how to maximise a player's fitness. A club, for example, will know how quickly each player recovers from different forms of exertion, how quickly he can run over ten yards, over 20 yards, how high he can jump...'

BORN TO PLAY FOOTBALL

Unlike other high intensity sports such as rugby – where the body shapes and sizes of players can vary enormously – footballers, generally-speaking, have similar physiques. Okay, so there might be a marginal height difference of 12 inches between Peter Crouch (6 feet 7 inches) and Lionel Messi (5 feet 7 inches) and don't forget football's legendary midget Diego Maradona, but on the whole footballers are similarly built.

Your average professional footballer weighs in at around 12 stone and is above average height of around 6 feet 2 inches. Sturdy enough to be able to hold his ground in a jostle for the ball, yet light enough to turn on a sixpence and move quickly around the park. Any heavier and, while players may very well be able to withstand the force of a flying headbutt from French force Zinedine Zidane and laugh at him nursing a sore head, the extra muscular or fatty bulk can result in loss of agility and competitive edge.

There is a very common misconception that top class footballers are rippling with muscles and spend hours in the gym growing their guns and chiselling away at their six-pack. In fact, as will be explained in more detail later, footballers spend relatively little training their upper body and instead spend most of it working on their skills and cardiovascular fitness.

So what can you do to give yourself the best possible physical conditioning to get anywhere close to the professionals? Actually, probably more than you think.

All top footballers will have been born with the perfect genes to play the game at the top level in terms of lung capacity and a high percentage of fast twitch muscle fibres but these attributes can be developed by anyone. Okay, so you might not have the time available to train as much as the top players and without the added incentive of £80k a week it isn't easy, but by integrating certain, highly-specific fitness drills into your workouts, you will be able to make the most of whatever genetic cards you were dealt at birth.

OPTIMISING POTENTIAL

Responsible for professional sportsmen who command a weekly wage that could virtually halve third world debt, the management and conditioning staff at every Premiership club expect their charges to justify their salary and produce the goods on the field.

Of course, every player has an off day – with England's

Paul Robinson's 'swing and miss' effort when he let in a howler against Croatia in 2006 being a memorable example – but if a player's form goes into steep decline due to a lack of fitness they can be shown the door pretty damn quick. Without exceptional conditioning and a body firing on all cylinders, players can be found wanting and on the transfer list if they do not stick to their side of the deal and give the club what they want, so it's in their interests to stay in shape both during and out of season.

Unlike your typical Sunday league club, who have a sole stalwart old chap – usually called Bill – to sponge bruised ankles and direct a few fitness drills, Premiership clubs have an army of fitness and conditioning staff constantly monitoring players and ensuring they eat properly and maintain the body composition which is expected of them. The key physical components which are checked frequently include:

- Body fat
- Cardiovascular fitness
- Flexibility
- Speed
- Strength

Let's take a look at each of these physiological attributes and see not only what effect they have on physical performance but also how the elite train specifically to optimise each component and how you can replicate it without all those physiologists and conditioning coaches.

BODY FAT

As an amateur player you may not think an extra stone here or there makes a significant difference to your game, but trust me: if you are carrying a few extra pounds from too many post-match kebabs and pints of Stella you'd see a massive difference in your game were you to lose the extra weight. Although there have been countless exceptions, such as gravity-defying Neville Southall, who despite carrying a few extra stone could jump around the goalmouth as energetically as Bambi on speed, if you lose fat your performance will improve dramatically – period.

Naturally, there's a big difference between carrying extra weight in the shape of muscle (which we'll discuss later) as opposed to fat, but if your physique is making people wonder whether it was actually you who ate some, if not all, the pies then I'd strongly suggest you read on and see what the pros do to make sure their body fat levels are at the optimum level to stay match fit – and just as vital, keep their coaches happy.

In a Premiership season, it's obviously in the players' interests to keep their body fat percentage in check (topless goal celebrations just don't look great with love handles), but after the season is over and players are not regularly monitored by their club's fitness and conditioning team, lack of training and accountability can lead to unwanted weight gain – and a major bollocking once pre-season training starts.

The senior conditioning coach of one club, which shall remain nameless, told me that one player reported in after their summer break carrying an excessive amount of extra body fat. During the four-week break, the player had packed on an extra 5 per cent body fat and whereas coaches will on the whole encourage players to take a break from the game and get some R-and-R between seasons, there are still certain rules which players must stick to in terms of body composition and fitness levels. Needless to say, an increase of 5 per cent body fat is excessive – and we'll be finding out exactly what that can mean later in this chapter.

Break the rules at your peril, as this particular player realised when he was fined a week's wages for putting on too much weight. Ironically, the fine was used to pay for a state-of-the-art gym at the club.

So, to ensure players can't get away with it, their body fat percentages are checked before, during and post-season to ensure their nutrition is correct and their bodies are able to perform at the maximum potential on the field.

A notable exception to this rule was legendary Sheffield United goal keeper William 'Fatty' Foulke, who tipped the scales at a staggering 24 stone. Although this was back in 1902 and the importance of body composition and its relationship with mobility and athleticism was clearly not as highly regarded as it is today, he can't have been that bad if he played top flight back then. The stories of Fatty Foulke's goal-keeping career are countless but one incident recalled by a linesman at one of his matches tells the story of Mr Foulke's anger at an equalising goal Southampton put past him in the dying minutes of the game which 'Fatty' had adjudged to be offside. After the match, Sheffield's tubby keeper remonstrated with the officials and stormed to the door of the referee's dressing room, clothed in nothing more than the suit he was born in. It's unclear whether the referee refused to come out due to the fear of a right hook or the unsavoury sight of a stark bollock-naked 24-stone man but, either way, the issue was resolved and Mr Foulke put some clothes on, much to the relief of the officials and his team-mates.

Over a century since Fatty Foulke's antics, the importance of body composition in performance sports is now regarded to be one of the most important factors in giving athletes that competitive edge and common sense tells you why.

Take a normal, every-day, recreational footballer who weighs in at 80 kg and enjoys a few post match beers and the occasional Meat Lovers pizza. Despite exercising and training two or three times a week, a sedentary job stuck behind a desk plus the cumulative effect of the weekend's beers and too many takeaways means his body fat level is 20 per cent.

So, at 20 per cent body fat, the total weight of fatty tissue being stored on his body is a staggering 16 kg. That's 16 bags of sugar, doing nothing more than weighing him down, making a 30 or 40 yard dash for the ball one hell of a lot harder than it should be.

Just a 5 per cent reduction in body fat would reduce the unnecessary baggage of our friend by 4 kg, making that sprint for the ball a lot easier, simply because he has 5 per cent less good-for-nothing weight to lug around.

At the top level of any sport, games and races are won by fractions of seconds and the slightest of margins, so it's hardly surprising that conditioning staff are incredibly strict about the amount of excess fat their players carry. Sir Clive Woodward, the manager of the English rugby team who won the 2003 World Cup, was famously quoted as saying the difference between a team winning and losing is doing 99 things just one per cent better than the opposition. And body fat percentage is one of those 'things'.

Players may very well get a bit narky at the pettiness of getting the riot act thrown at them for putting on just 2 per cent of body fat, but at the elite level 2 per cent is a significant amount of weight. Coaching staff see that as an extra bag or two of sugar tied around the waist of a player for 90 minutes and know very well that they stand a far better chance of getting to the ball first or lasting the 90 minutes were it not there.

These days, when players are given contracts they all know the rules about maintaining pre-determined body fat levels and know they have to stay within the limits, but what if they stray? And what can be done to get their body fat percentage back down to acceptable limits?

As I highlighted earlier, in the first instance most players are fined a week's wages for getting too chubby and often a sound talking-to is enough to get them back on side (so to speak) and clean up their act. After a dressing down, a range of steps are then taken to shed the extra fat and get players back to an optimal playing weight.

Consultations with the club nutritionist, fitness coaches and even psychologists address the reasons why body fat levels have exceeded normal levels and, working as a team, they may devise a six-to-eight-week programme to ensure the player's training, diet and state of mind is refocused. Reassessments are then made after the six-to-eight weeks, sometimes more frequently and, assuming all is well, the player will be off the hook – for now.

FAT LOSS TIPS FOR RECREATIONAL PLAYERS

As a casual player, you have both an advantage and disadvantage over your Premiership counterparts. On the plus side, unless you have a coach who's a distant relative of Hitler and has the time, inclination and dictatorial instinct to keep tabs on your body fat levels, you are not really accountable to anyone for putting on a few pounds. The vast majority of lower league clubs who struggle for resources generally only have time to concentrate on ball skills and general fitness, leaving the more subtle aspects of conditioning – such as core strength and body composition – down to the individual. However, it is this lack of accountability which makes it very difficult to have the discipline to be conscientious about good nutrition and specific training to reduce unwanted body fat.

If you play recreationally or even semi-competitively and are concerned about the amount of body fat you are carrying, your first job is to calculate your body fat percentage. There are a number of ways you can do this but a fitness instructor at your local gym should be able to give you a pretty accurate reading. This is explained in more detail in chapter two.

The chances are, assuming that you lead a moderately active lifestyle, at the same time enjoying the occasional evening with your friends Stella and Artois, your body fat percentage will be somewhere in the region of 15-20 per cent.

To put this figure into some kind of perspective, as a rough guide, Premiership footballers possess a body fat level of around 10 per cent which may fluctuate to a degree during the off season but will certainly not go any higher than 12 per cent. On the opposite end of the scale, to be classed as clinically obese your body fat level needs to rise to 30 per cent, at which point your doctor will persuade you to do something about it.

So, assuming you sit somewhere between those extremes and have a body fat level of about 20 per cent and want to do something about it to improve your game, you have to consider three things:

1 How much fat do I want to lose?
2 How much of a lifestyle change am I willing to embrace?
3 How realistic is it that I'll meet my goal?

It's very easy to sit back and think to yourself, Right, I'm going to lose 10 per cent of my body fat and be as cut as Ronaldo... but is this realistic?

You've got to remember that these guys have every resource they need, from nutritionists who will tell them exactly what and how much they should be eating to fitness specialists who will tell them exactly the right amount of exercise to do to help maintain (and improve) performance while at the same time burn away their excess body fat. What many people do not realise is that this sort of advice is not just a generic eating or fitness plan printed off the computer and given to the chubby footballer but a programme designed specifically for that individual player.

Every person on this planet and every player who plays competitive football (to whatever level) is metabolically different and responds in their own way to various methods of training stimuli and nutrition, so a one-size-fits-all approach is as useful as a chocolate teapot.

As an amateur you have to settle with using your own initiative and self-discipline to bring your body fat levels down. First of all you need to assess how much you are willing to change your lifestyle in order to meet your goal.

To help you do this, here are some very simple facts which you must consider before declaring war on your love handles.

- One kilogram of fat contains 9000 calories
- A large doner kebab can contain more than a thousand calories
- A pint of lager contains around 150 calories
- A mile run at a steady pace will burn off about a hundred calories

Well, there was no point in deluding you. Exercise has to go together with sensible eating.

Losing fat is not easy, but it is essential you take a realistic look at your lifestyle and make a decision on how much you are willing to change it rather than setting yourself an unrealistic goal destined for failure.

After taking in those facts you might be undecided about whether you can, after all, actually be bothered to go to war with your excess baggage. But before you become completely disheartened by the task, take a look at the positives: a few months of hard work will leave you more attractive to the opposite sex (or same sex depending on your persuasion), you'll feel so much better about yourself and, more importantly, you will see a staggering improvement in your performance on the football field.

Cynical? Don't be.

The following table is the result of some in-depth research into the effect of body fat on a selection of performance tests. This study was carried out over a series of three trials on three groups of men, who were classified into 3 levels of 'fatness' – low, moderate and high.

The results speak for themselves:

LEVEL OF FATNESS AS PERCENTAGE OF BODY FAT

Test	Low <10 per cent	Moderate <10-15 per cent	High >15 per cent
75-yard dash (es)	9.8	10.1	10.7
220-yard dash (es)	29.3	31.6	35.0
Standing long jump (feet)	23.8	22.7	20.2
Sit-ups in two minutes	43.4	41.6	36.2

The number of sit-ups performed in two minutes is largely irrelevant but the significance of the dash test and standing jump are hugely insightful to any athlete or footballer – whatever standard.

So whether you play for Chelsea or Accrington Stanley,

the facts are there to see – the more useless blubber you can shift from your body the faster you'll run and the higher you'll jump. All you've got to do now is to dedicate the off season to addressing the issue and work hard at burning off the lard.

What is the best way to go about it without the luxury of your own personal nutritionist and conditioning coach?

There are a number of ways to get your body fat levels down and depending on your own genetic make-up and mind-set, the speed and ease it takes you to get that body fat percentage down can vary enormously.

The best suggestion is to spend a little money on a consultation with a well-qualified personal trainer who will be able not only to analyse your body fat levels but will also look at your physique, analyse your diet and make some sound and realistic suggestions on how best to achieve your goal.

If you don't have the luxury of spare funds for a personal trainer then you should keep things simple. Stick to the following basic principles – which are not far off those followed by the pros – and you'll be amazed at how quickly you will see results.

KEEP A FOOD DIARY

Although it can be a bit of an arse having to write down everything that passes your lips, keeping a food diary for a week or more is a great way of seeing where you are going wrong and where you are consuming excessive and unnecessary calories. It's amazing how easy and frequently the odd chocolate bar or packet of crisps can creep into your diet and just how quickly the calories add up during a week of snacky and fatty foods.

After a week or so of keeping a food diary you'll be able to pick out where you are going wrong and what foods you should be eliminating from your diet to give yourself the best chance to shed those unnecessary pounds.

REGULAR EXERCISE

It's not difficult to work out that, in order to shift what is effectively stored energy, you need to train to burn it off and expend it. The trouble many people have when it comes to exercising for fat loss is that they don't know how hard they should train, how regularly they should train or what sort of training they should be doing.

As a footballer, the one single form of exercise you will be doing most on the pitch is run. Therefore, why not do what the pros do and kill two birds with one stone by basing your fitness training and fat burning exercise around running?

However, by running I do not mean setting off for a gentle jog trotting along at a comfortable pace; I mean pushing yourself hard through a series of shuttle runs running at around 85 per cent of your maximum effort and feeling exhausted by the end of it.

High intensity running, as you'll read later, is an essential component of football fitness and benefits the body in a number of ways:

● It makes the body secrete growth hormone, a key
  hormone which melts away body fat

- It elevates your resting metabolic rate for longer than low intensity exercise, meaning that your body will be burning off fat for up to 48 hours after training
- It conditions the fast twitch muscle fibres in the legs, making you a more efficient and faster runner
- It strengthens your heart and cardiovascular system to be better able to tolerate the demands of the game

Losing body fat, whether you're a footballer or couch potato is never easy, but once you get your mind-set right, reducing the size of your love handles becomes a far easier mountain to climb.

There are countless elite players who have struggled with weight over the years but with the right incentives and, luckily for them, the right conditioning coaches, getting down to a more competitive weight has turned around their careers.

Do not underestimate the importance of your level of body fat and your ability to play the game and play it well. If you are still unconvinced and reckon you could play just as well with or without a beer belly, you might want to consider buying a weighted jacket which fits around your torso and can weigh up to eight kilograms. Try training or even playing in that for 90 minutes and then tell me the extra dead weight doesn't weigh you down and make you feel knackered after just half-an-hour.

CARDIOVASCULAR TRAINING
Few people can argue that Premiership footballers train exceptionally hard to achieve the high fitness levels required to play week in, week out at such high intensities.

However, very few people actually know exactly how they adapt their heart and lungs to tear around the pitch at high speeds for 90 minutes. It's not simply a case of going out for a quick run every now and again; these guys have world-class sports scientists and fitness coaches who design highly specific training regimes so that the players are conditioned correctly for the game. True, they might have the ideal genes for tearing around a football pitch and a natural talent for rolling around in apparent agony when they get a hurty knee, but they still have to train exceptionally hard to maximise their fitness potential.

It has been demonstrated in a number of studies that top-class centre forwards will run over a mile during a match at a very high intensity at speeds exceeding 20 kilometres an hour and at speeds of closer to 25 kilometres an hour for around one kilometre.

This level of running intensity demonstrates to anyone interested in improving their football fitness the importance of training hard to adapt their body to the requirements of a game. A five-mile steady jog just doesn't cut the mustard.

CARDIOVASCULAR SECRETS REVEALED

A lot of the best parts of cardiovascular training programmes at the top clubs have been kept under wraps – until now.

I have gained exclusive access to a top Premiership fitness coach and pushed him to reveal a few of the tips and trick that the pros use to make them the human version of the Duracell Bunny. The details of some of these training regimes are covered in the next chapter but to gain an understanding why players train in a certain way, it's important to learn a little bit about the physiology first and why players have to certain forms of training to make them the athletes that they are.

In order to help a footballer reach his full potential, his heart, lungs and legs muscles need to be trained correctly to give him maximum impact on the field. This is done in a number of ways but, cardiovascularly, his body needs to be pushed through three different types of 'energy systems' at certain points of pre-season training to ensure his explosive speed and speed endurance is at a peak when the season starts. Despite already possessing these physiological attributes through his genetic make-up, his cardiovascular system still has to be honed to match or exceed that of other players.

The following explanations of the different training intensities that the elite players run at to condition their bodies will give you a very good idea about what forms of training they do and how you can mimic them to achieve a level of fitness you have only ever dreamed of.

The three training intensities, or systems, that the top Premiership coaches will make their players work at are known as the:

- Aerobic system
- Lactate system
- Creatine phosphate system

I'm not going to go into detail explaining the in-depth science behind these training systems, but for the good of your own training and to serve as an insight as to what the pros do, the following explanations should give you a good overview.

AEROBIC TRAINING

Generally speaking, all exercise performed at a steady state, such as walking or jogging, is classed as aerobic exercise.

Aerobic exercise is fuelled by the oxidation of fats and carbohydrates by using the oxygen we breathe in. At this intensity the body is easily able to take in, transport and utilise oxygen and supply it to the working muscles in sufficient amounts so that the energy sources (predominantly carbohydrate and fat) can be oxidised and used to fuel movement.

As a footballer all this is, of course, essential but spending excessive time in conditioning your aerobic capacity by embarking on long-distance, medium-paced runs is not conducive to a 90-minute game of football. Although a certain degree of aerobic training is of use to any footballer, particularly at the beginning of pre-season training, when it can be used to waken the heart and leg muscles after time off, its performance benefits are minimal when taken to the extreme.

Think about it. During a match, the key emphasis on a player's fitness has to be on his ability to withstand repeated bouts of high intensity running at near maximum speed with only short breaks. He should be able to run around for the whole 90 minutes and be in good enough shape to cover 8-12 kilometres in the process, but it's a waste of training time if excessive hours are spent going for long distance runs performed at a steady pace. That's not what you do when you play football, so why train like it?

So, when your pre-season training involves you jogging along with a mate and you have enough breath to talk about your plans for a few beers on the weekend – you are not working properly. If you are serious about your football and really want to get anywhere close to the fitness levels of the Premiership elite, ditch your casual, low-intensity jogs and concentrate on the fat-burning, lung-busting lactate training instead.

However, there is one aspect of aerobic training which is of great importance and interest to Premiership fitness coaches. They may not give a monkey's that you can jog along aerobically at 70 per cent of your maximum speed for three hours but they do want to know what your maximum aerobic capacity is – also known as 'VO2 max'.

The term VO2 max is often over-used by part-time fitness coaches who in truth don't actually have a clue what it means. I have spoken to dozens of aspiring football players over the years who use the term 'VO2 max' in the most random of ways. I'm left not only wondering what the hell they are talking about but where they got their information from.

A player's VO2 max can be best described as: '*The maximum amount of oxygen a player can take in, transport and utilise*'.

So what does this mean in layman's terms?

Put simply, your VO2 max is the peak value of your aerobic capacity and a general indicator of your cardiovascular fitness. You reach your VO2 max when you train to the point at which you cannot physically take in more oxygen to supply to your leg muscles.

It is expressed in ml/kg/min. Or in plain English: *millilitres (of oxygen) per kilogram (of body weight) per minute (of work performed)*.

Your maximal oxygen uptake (VO2 max) will be reached when you are working very close to your maximum heart rate (HR max), so when you are at or very close to exercising at your maximum capacity, it can be said that you are training at your VO2 max. This level of work can obviously only be performed for a short period of time before fatigue sets in, lactic acid overwhelms your muscles and you collapse in a heap.

It must be made clear that understanding or knowing your own VO2 max is not an essential part of football training for the majority of amateur players but it may be of interest to some interested in exercise physiology and optimal performance. Unfortunately for the game's elite there is no escaping regular VO2 max tests for them and they are dreaded by all players – except those who love pain and the overwhelming desire to see their lunch again. VO2 max tests are hard but they do give the conditioning staff a lot of information about both a player's physical fitness and their mental strength to push their bodies to the limit.

I will go into more detail about exactly how the Premiership stars' VO2 max levels are assessed in the next chapter. Many of you may very well already have undertaken a VO2 max assessment at your club in the form of the bleep test (where you perform a series of shuttle runs between markers 20 metres apart). Although a fairly dated form of VO2 max testing, it is still of value and many of the top clubs will still use it from time to time to gauge players' fitness levels.

SIZE IS NOT EVERYTHING

Even highly competent fitness coaches can get caught up in the scientific value of a player's VO2 max. It is worth pointing out that a player with a high VO2 max does not necessarily have a superior level of fitness compared with a runner with a lower VO2 max. Although the ability to take in, transport and utilise more oxygen than a competitor may appear to be an advantage, studies suggest that some athletes are able to maintain exercise at a higher percentage of their VO2 max than someone with a higher VO2 max.

A perfect example of this is the former marathon world-record holder Alberto Salazar who had a recorded VO2 max of 70ml/kg/min (which is good but not great). Experts were baffled and suggested his marathon time of 2 hours 6 minutes should result in a much higher VO2 max. It was discovered that he was beating his rivals, all with far superior VO2 max levels, because he was able to maintain a running speed at an impressive 86 per cent of VO2 max.

To put all this in perspective, elite footballers have been shown to have VO2 max levels in the range of 55-70ml/kg/min. To date the highest-recorded maximum oxygen uptake is that of a cross-country skier who was recorded to have a VO2 max of a massive 94ml/kg/min.

Whether you wish to regularly review your VO2 max status or just check up on it every now and again, remember to keep all the figures and terms in perspective. You may have an impressive VO2 max but in the dying minutes of a game when your legs are burning and you are exhausted, mental strength overtakes maximal oxygen uptake as a means to keep your composure and not succumb to your physical fatigue.

LACTATE TRAINING (ANAEROBIC TRAINING)
Now we're talking.

Conditioning the body to tolerate high levels of lactic acid in the body is vital for performance and really sorts the men from the boys. It's what the pros spend a lot of time doing, in a number of different ways, in the run up to a season and when you look at what the training involves, it's not difficult to see why it is so important.

There is no reason why you can't copy the examples of lactate training outlined in chapter three to help improve your fitness. Just because the likes of Rooney, Terry and Walcott might do the sessions faster and with fewer and shorter breaks, it's all relative and with time you'll be way ahead of the game in terms of fitness.

Many people who train on their own find it hard to know not only how to train their lactate system properly but also how long and how frequently they should train. The good news for most of you who already play for a club and are put through a series of vomit-inducing, pre-season training sessions is that your fitness coach will make you train your lactate system without you really knowing about it.

The terms lactate and lactic acid are often confused as the same thing but technically they are slightly different. If you really want to know, lactic acid is an acid and lactate is an acid salt but going into detail about this is best left to the biology textbooks.

When players train their lactate system, they are essentially pushing themselves to intensity where the body is unable to breathe in sufficient amounts of oxygen and supply it to the muscles.

If exercise is to continue, the body needs to find energy from other sources. In this case, it breaks down stored carbohydrate and converts it into a usable form of energy which is then utilised by the leg muscles to keep motoring.

When training in this 'anaerobic state' (without oxygen), there are consequences. A burst of instant, explosive energy is paid for in the form of oxidative by-products which the muscles are unable to tolerate in high quantities. Lactic acid is the main result which you will be aware of – because you will doubtless have experienced the agony it puts you in.

If lactic acid levels rise too high, your leg muscles will start to burn and in most cases you feel nauseous – hence the reason you want to throw up during a particularly nasty pre-season training session.

Depending on your individual level of tolerance and fitness levels, lactic acid has a huge impact on your performance, as its presence in your muscles simply makes it impossible for them to contract at their maximum capacity. This results in a dramatic drop in speed, making the difference between racing in defence to make a match-saving tackle or slowing down your approach to goal.

On a positive note, as menacing as lactic acid is, it is possible to make your body adapt and condition it to be more able to cope with high levels in the blood stream and also be able to get rid of it quicker. As the lactate system is trained, the nauseous feeling tends to subside and you are able to tolerate more abuse from your coach.

So how can you tell if you are training your lactate system?

Put simply, once the intensity of a run increases to a level of about 90 per cent of your maximum pace – where your ability to talk has virtually gone, you have to really concentrate on what you are doing and you feel your thighs start to burn after about 60 seconds – then you can assume that you are working your lactate system.

Very unfit people may only be able to put up with 30 seconds of running at 90 per cent of their maximum pace before collapsing in a heap, whereas top-conditioned Premiership footballers could quite happily (a loose term) function at this intensity for well over 60 seconds.

The good news is that you don't have to be a Premiership superstar with an army of sports science boffins to help you improve your tolerance to lactic acid. With sufficient and specific training, it is possible to build up a tolerance to perform exercise at these intensities, helping to significantly improve repeated explosive sprints and delaying the time before fatigue sets in. Repeated high-intensity sprints with very little rest might not sound like your idea of fun, but they'll do wonders for helping you build up a tolerance to lactic acid in your muscles.

CREATINE PHOSPHATE SYSTEM

The creatine phosphate system is an instant energy system which is used by the body for short, high-intensity activities such as sprinting and jumping. Whenever you see players do an all-out sprint or perform a gazelle-like leap into the air it means the creatine phosphate energy system is in use. It must be conditioned properly to utilise its full potential and the elite will spend one heck of a lot of time honing this system to ensure they are explosive around the park.

This system is pretty easy to understand and, in principle, also straightforward to condition. Put simply, whenever your muscles need instant energy for a fast and explosive muscular contraction, the body injects the muscles with a chemical called creatine phosphate. This chemical has a similar effect to gushes of fuel in those engine injector systems found in certain cars, but unfortunately it is in limited supply.

To illustrate this perfectly, perform standing jumps as high as you can. You might be able to do five or six at a maximal effort but after that your muscles start to get tired and you find you start to lose height. Keep going, and you'll start to accumulate lactic acid and then the lactate system kicks in.

The creatine phosphate system typically gives you just five to eight seconds of instant energy before stores are depleted and performance starts to go downhill, so for footballers it's vital to train this system. At the same time you will train fast twitch muscle fibres – more on these later

– to increase intramuscular creatine stores and make your short, explosive sprints that much quicker. You'll also delay the onset of lactic acid.

If you are into your supplements and already take your training seriously, you may well have come across the supplement creatine monohydrate in health food stores. I'll go into more detail about supplemental creatine later and how, besides resistance-training and conditioning those fast twitch muscle fibres to tolerate high intensity movements more effectively, there are a few nutritional and supplemental secrets which the pros, and you, can use legally to really kick some proverbial ass.

FLEXIBILITY

Of all the fitness attributes required to play football, flexibility is often way down on the list of priorities for the amateur footballer and it's not difficult to see why.

Spending a good 15 to 20 minutes – let alone an hour like the pros – warming up the major leg and trunk muscles is pretty dull when there are a dozen-odd footballs out on the pitch ready to be kicked around. It's a classic sight at all lower league clubs: players come out of the dressing room and the first thing they do is run up to a ball and hoof it the 40 yards towards a keeperless goalmouth.

Despite being the perfect way to rip your hamstring muscles, this approach before a game is embedded in the psyche of most players and is very difficult to change. I have witnessed many a conscientious player start with good intentions and stretch a quad or two before a severe case of

FOMO (Fear of Missing Out) overwhelms them and they join their mates for a kick-around.

This, however, is at Sunday league level. In top-flight professional football, if a player so much as looks at a ball before warming up properly the conditioning staff and coach will make sure the football(s) is rammed right up where the sun don't shine.

Flexibility training and stretching before a game or practice is an integral part of physical preparation and its importance should not be underestimated by players of any level.

The Premiership has seen a significant shift in attitude towards flexibility training in the last decade, in part due to major advances in using stretching and flexibility techniques to prevent injury and even improve performance. Some teams employ a stretching specialist to assist the physiotherapy team and the conditioning staff to ensure each player is rehabilitated or conditioned optimally so that their price tag can be utilised on the pitch rather than on the physio's bench.

However, this is not to say that all Premierships players are flexible. In fact, many players have been found to have a lower than average level of flexibility due to the fact that players' muscles constantly contract during training and playing and so have a preponderance to tighten up.

The trouble with flexibility training and pre- and post-match stretching is that it is not particularly interesting. Despite playing at the top level, players are notoriously poorly disciplined at stretching out tight muscles and conditioning staff are forever nagging players to stretch.

WHY ARE FLEXIBILITY AND STRETCHING SO IMPORTANT?

Some people are lucky when it comes to flexibility. We all know someone who has a party trick where they can do the splits or bend over backwards without preparation in a move which would snap most people's spines. This ability, to a large part, is down to genetics.

Some players are lucky and possess a naturally high level of flexibility, however most players need to work at it for the good of their game and resistance to injury.

As with the cardiovascular training, I could carp on about the importance of flexibility but for the purposes of this book I'll just cover the essentials and tell you how stretching can make you a better player. Many Premiership players whinge and moan about following a flexibility programme but those who comply with the fitness staff often spend far less time nursing pulled muscles and more time scoring goals.

So what benefits does a regular stretching and flexibility routine have on a player apart from making him more bendy? Probably more than you think. Decades of research into the science of stretching has discovered the following benefits:

- Improves range of movement in the joints
- Reduces muscular tension
- Significantly reduces the chances of contracting muscular strains and joint sprains
- Reduces the chances of suffering from back pain – a major problem for many footballers
- Helps to reduce muscle soreness after a game.

- Decreases the viscosity of the muscles, which helps to ensure that the muscle fibres slide smoothly.
- Improves posture, which is essential for a fully functional athlete.

If I had to highlight the one area where Premiership footballers had to dedicate more time, flexibility training would be at the top of the list.

None of the benefits listed above are exaggerated. I have travelled to America as a trainer on a number of occasions to attend injury rehabilitation and biomechanics seminars, lectures and courses which all highlighted the significance of stretching for the longevity of a professional sportsman's career. It's an aspect of your training, even as a non-professional player, which you can really improve on.

STRETCHING AND COMMON INJURIES

Premiership footballers may very well have the perfect combination of genes to make them skilful, fast and strong but their flexibility is often compromised due to these very attributes.

Even as a casual player, this will also be the case with you.

All those years ago, back when you were in nappies and did nothing all day other than eat, poop and cry, your flexibility was awesome. My own daughter currently has a fascination with sucking her toes, which she chews on without being in any discomfort whatsoever. Why? Well the fascination with her toes I'm not sure about but, as someone who isn't yet able to walk, her muscles are fairly idle.

However, as soon as more muscular activity is introduced and they contract and relax under tension to initiate movement, the muscles will begin to tighten and become less flexible.

Now take this to the other extreme and look at the top players whose vigorous training regimes and game time involves their muscles contracting thousands and thousands of times a day, causing them to shorten and tighten. Unless these muscles are stretched regularly the increased tightness can lead to a range of injuries – from back pain to repeated hamstring tears. We're specifically looking at leg muscles here, though it's true of other groups as well.

To illustrate my point and give you a real life example of how stretching can help reduce back problems and torn hamstrings, consider the following cases which are typical of all high performance sportsmen – not just footballers. By understanding the following cases, you'll gain a good insight into how tight muscles can adversely affect the body and how you can prevent the same happening to you.

TORN HAMSTRINGS

Most footballers have had a hamstring tweak at sometime. You sprint after a ball and all of a sudden you feel a sharp pain in the back of your leg and running any further is either painful or near impossible.

Hamstrings can commonly 'go' after they are put under a massive amount of strain, usually when accelerating. The increased tension in the muscle is not able to cope with the force. So, like a stiff rubber band being pulled too hard, it snaps. Of course, there are varying degrees of hamstring tear – from the ripping of just a few fibres to extreme cases when the entire muscle snaps – and you can, literally, hear it snap!

More often than not, hamstring tears happen for one of two reasons:

1 The muscles are not warmed up properly and due to the fact that they act like Plasticine and snap if they are cold, any aggressive or sudden movement can make them ping.
2 Despite being warm, the muscles are so tight that they are under constant tension. To a degree this is good. It is this tension which contributes to fast leg speed – but if they are too tight they are more susceptible to tearing when under tension.

As with nearly all the tips in this book, the Premiership stars have the fitness and physio teams constantly keeping an eye on every player's level of flexibility and, although it might be difficult to make them stretch on their own, if need be they will be regularly stretched by a physiotherapist. As for you, unless you are fortunate enough to be able to afford to pay for regular visits to the physio, you are going to need the discipline to stretch yourself.

BACK PAIN
As back pain and, specifically, low back pain (LBP) are among the most common causes of discomfort in both the sedentary

and active population, this section of the book could go on forever.

Back pain in footballers is also common, but rarely so severe to prevent playing. The wonder of pain killers and massage therapy can keep most problems at bay but their persistence can leave players pretty fed up and pissed off a lot of the time.

The trouble with back pain is the difficulty in locating one specific cause. Soft tissue damage, disc hernia, inflammation, ligament sprains and muscle tears can all lead to players injuring their backs, but often prevention is far simpler than you may think. By addressing muscular imbalances through regular stretching, you can cure back pain incredibly quickly and more often than not, the services of that physio will no longer be needed.

Perhaps the best example of this is the tightening of the hip flexor muscles.

Among all the actions that footballers do a lot, it's safe to say that running is at the top of the list. Running for several hours a day, week in, week out, uses an array of leg muscles, and a major group is called hip flexors. These are positioned at the front of the pelvis and their action moves the thighs upward – that movement repeatedly performed in running.

As explained earlier, repeated muscular contraction causes muscles to shorten and over time this shortening can have a pulling effect on the pelvis, put it under tension and, in some cases, even cause it to tilt forwards. This tension can have a knock-on effect for a number of other muscles which attach to the pelvis and put them under strain – in most cases when this happens, it is the back which can become inflamed and sore.

As you can see, biomechanically, it's not a difficult concept to grasp and easy to see how such a simple case of a shortened muscle has effects elsewhere in the body.

In this instance, as soon as the diagnosis is made, a series of simple stretches for excessively short hip flexors can help to fix the problem and football can be resumed without any nagging back pain.

As you can see from these two examples, you cannot over-estimate the importance of stretching. It might be a ball-ache to do and, in the large part, pretty dull, but keeping your muscles flexible can make a dramatic impact to your game and prevent a range of injury from muscle tears to back pain

Of course, some players are lucky to possess the genes which result in a naturally good level of flexibility, regardless of how much high intensity training they do, but sadly most of us need to be disciplined and stretch regularly.

MUSCLE MAKE UP AND SPEED – IT'S ALL ABOUT THE FIBRES

Did you know that...

- The human body contains over 600 muscles, nine controlling the thumb alone?
- A muscle fibre's use of energy can be over 200 times more during exercise than at rest?

Do you remember all those years ago when you were at school and on Sports Day there were always a handful of your classmates who excelled in one event or another? The same faces did well every year at the 100-metre sprint and invariably, but not always, another group of your peers would excel at the longer distances.

At such a young age, these differences in sporting ability did not arise through intensive, sports-specific training but due to the genetic 'cards' each individual was dealt when they were born.

A number of variances in genetic make-up can help to contribute to athletic success but the differences in muscle fibre plays a significant role in whether an individual excels in explosive events or longer-duration, endurance events.

The explosive, breakneck speed at which top flight football is played clearly demonstrates that in order to play game at the top level you need to have pace – and lots of it. Once again, even though most players possess a natural ability to run fast, highly specific training can make them faster.

To give you an idea of what happens at a physiological level, I thought it would be helpful to give you an insight into how the muscles are conditioned to achieve optimum speed and maximise potential.

When it comes down to the muscles themselves, different types of fibres are called upon, according to the intensity of exercise being performed.

Our musculature is generally made up of two different types of muscle fibre and are either classed as 'slow twitch' or 'fast twitch' type I and II.

As their name suggests, slow twitch fibres contract relatively slowly and are used for activities which require less explosive movements – such as endurance running. Marathon runners have a high percentage of slow twitch fibres.

Fast twitch fibres contract rapidly and are called upon for activities that require fast movements, such as sprinting. Needless to say, it is the fast twitch fibres which you must focus on to make significant fitness gains.

Studies of identical twins have proved that the ratio of muscle fibres we possess is genetically predetermined, suggesting that even before we have taken our first step our inherited muscle fibre ratio means we are destined to excel in one sport or another. However, just because someone is born with a higher ratio of slow twitch muscle fibres does not necessarily mean that they will be unsuccessful at competing in high-speed events. With sufficient training, research suggests that one fibre type can take on the characteristics of the opposite type.

So, just because you are slow it does not mean that you are destined to be slow forever. With the right training – described later – you can increase your speed immeasurably.

FAST TWITCH MUSCLE FIBRES

Of the two types of fast twitch fibres, it is type II which is responsible for that explosive burst of pace.

When a sudden sprint is initiated, it is your fast twitch muscles that are recruited to work, due to their ability to generate creatine phosphate (CP) at a quicker rate. At an all-out sprint, they are used at full capacity, not only because of their ability to produce CP but also because of the speed at which fast twitch fibres are able to contract.

For players, both at the top and at Sunday league level, training fast-twitch muscle fibres is essential part of pre-season training to help improve speed and explosive movements such as jumping and lunging for the ball.

HEART RATE AND LUNG CAPACITY

Here are some facts about your heart and lungs which may surprise you:

- The heart is responsible for circulating the blood through around 60,000 miles (100,000 kilometres) of blood vessels
- The resting heart rate of a supremely fit Premiership footballer can be as low as 35 beats per minute, compared to 80 beats per minute of someone who only exercises occasionally
- The heart beats around 35,000,000 times a year (100,000 times a day)
- The heart pumps about 14,000 litres (3,600 gallons) of blood around the body every day
- During a run, the amount of gas passing in and out of the lungs (pulmonary ventilation) can vary from 120 litres per minute in untrained runners up to a massive 240 litres per minute in highly trained athletes
- The maximum amount of oxygen that can be inhaled, transported and utilised in the body (VO2max) can vary

from 40 millilitres per kilogram of body weight per minute (40ml/kg/min) in untrained runners to 77ml/kg/min in world class athletes

● Your left lung is approximately ten per cent smaller than your right lung

● The alveoli, which are responsible for gaseous exchange, have a surface area of around 70 square metres – about the size of a volley ball court

THE HEART

About the size of a fist, the heart is the 'biological pump' that supplies oxygenated blood to working muscles. The more work you ask of your muscles whilst running, the more your heart needs to beat in order to provide the muscles with a sufficient supply of nutrient-rich blood.

The hearts of top footballers are highly muscular and are able to pump vast quantities of blood to the working muscles very quickly. Without this ability, the Ronaldos of this world would look like very ordinary players and be blowing after just a 60-metre dash for the ball.

The amount of blood your heart ejects every beat is called stroke volume (SV) and the figure will depend on your fitness levels at the start of your training.

Subjects	SV at rest (ml)	SV (ml) during maximal exercise
Untrained/unfit player	55-75	80-110
Trained/reasonably	80-90	130-150
Premiership player	100-120	160-220 >

Table taken from Physiology of Sport and Exercise, *Costill and Wilmore, Human Kinetics Europe Ltd, 2005*

Stroke volume is low in untrained players simply because the heart has insufficient musculature and therefore isn't strong enough to pump large amounts of blood with each beat. As a result, the heart needs to beat faster to make up for the low stroke volume if the energy needs of the muscles are to be met. This is the main reason why unconditioned players who have either been off injured or taken a complete break from any training have a higher running heart rate than players who are in shape.

To make your heart adapt to the rigours of the game you need to perform a series of high intensity training runs – effectively, weight-training for your heart.

STRENGTH

Physical strength is relatively low down on the list of all the physical attributes required to play football at the top level and is a genetic characteristic which is not nearly as essential as high speed and good maximal cardiovascular capacity.

While strength in any sport is essential and there is a general belief that if you make an athlete 10 per cent stronger, he or she will be vastly more competitive, Premiership fitness coaches do not prioritise weight training over running drills when it comes to conditioning. Unlike sports like rugby where contact and aggressive tackling is an integral part of the game, football does not require such a focus on brute upper body strength and as ripped as the elite might look when they perform topless goal celebrations their strength is not what it appears. Their low levels of body fat may make their pecs and abs look impressive but do not fall for the belief that they have spent hours in the gym performing 30 kilogram dumbbell flies.

That said, players should not avoid upper body resistance training. In recent years, Premiership fitness coaches have come to recognise the benefits that a little bit of extra upper body strength can have when winning the ball in a one-on-one situation. Defender and striker often find themselves running shoulder-to-shoulder and a significant strength advantage can mean the difference between winning the ball and watching it disappear.

As an amateur player who has limited resources, the amount of time you dedicate to upper body strength training will understandably be low on your own list of fitness priorities but try to integrate a few basic strengthening exercises in your running drills. More is explained in chapter 3 on how exactly to do this.

CHAPTER TWO
PRE-SEASON AND FITNESS TESTING
CONDITIONING SECRETS
OF THE PROS

'Some people might think we are lazy, but that's fine. What's the point of tearing players to pieces in the first few days? We never bothered with sand dunes and hills and roads; we trained on grass, where football is played.'

Bill Shankly on pre-season training

It could never be said that Bill Shankly was one to mince his words at any point in his managerial career – even if he was sometimes a little wide of the mark. One of his classics came just before Liverpool took on West Ham in 1971 when he said to Kevin Keegan: 'Christ, son, I've just seen that Bobby Moore. What a wreck. He's got bags under his eyes, he's limping, he's got dandruff and it looks as if he has been to a nightclub again.'

Predictably, Moore played a blinder.

But when it comes to fitness training, Shankly's frank

opinion on pre-season is one which is echoed by a significant number of top fitness coaches in the league today. Although at one time it was almost fashionable to train up and down sand dunes and sprint up steep hills to train the legs, the view now taken is that this type of training is not specific enough for footballers and may even be detrimental to performance. All aspects of the game today, especially training, are looked at from a very scientific point of view and hills are pretty much viewed as a waste of training time.

'It's just not biomechanically specific enough for a stop-start game lasting 90 minutes on a flat pitch,' argues a top Premiership fitness coach.

FITNESS TESTING THE PREMIERSHIP WAY

Although there are always a handful of players at every club who have a masochistic love of the sheer agony of fitness testing, it is one aspect of pre-season that the majority of players dread. Ball skills and drills are generally a good laugh and a great chance to have some decent banter with your mates, but when it comes to lung-busting fitness testing, it can swiftly wipe the smile off the faces of even the most jovial squad members.

The pain of being pushed beyond your physical limits, often to the point of vomiting, might very well give your fitness coach an idea about how much off season training you have done and what sort of shape you're in but let's face it for most of us a weekend with the mother-in-law seems painless by comparison.

However, as nasty as it is, whatever your playing standard,

fitness testing is a vital part of the game and can tell you and your coach one hell of a lot about your physical condition and what aspects of fitness you need to work on in order to maximise your playing potential. It's all very well spending the summer on the beach practising your keepy-uppies, but fancy ball skills are not a lot of good if you are struggling to keep pace with the game.

Love it or hate it, if you want to get the most out of your season and maximise your skill levels, it is essential that you first find out how fit you are and then address your fitness shortfalls once they have been discovered.

When that time comes around for your pre-season fitness test and you're thinking of ways to cry off it, count yourself lucky that most clubs will only make you do it once – twice at worst – during a season. Fitness testing for your Premiership counterparts is an integral part of both pre- and mid-season training to ensure every player has the physicality to compete at the top level.

Although all clubs are different and all vary in the way they keep tabs on the fitness levels of their players, most scientifically monitor each player's fitness levels at least three times a year – more if players show signs of a drop in performance or after a chronic injury.

Of course, the advantage the players and the fitness staff have over you and your team manager is the availability of some serious laboratory gadgets which can analyse and calculate a huge amount of data from a player simply running on a treadmill and determine how well-conditioned their body is for a full 90 minutes of Premiership football.

Thanks to some contacts, I have managed to gain an insight into some of the fitness testing protocols performed at top Premiership clubs.

THE MEDICAL

Before contracts are officially exchanged or money changes hands on a new player, he must undergo a thorough physical examination to make sure he is not only cardiovascularly fit but also structurally sound. The fitness team and management need to be confident that any player coming to the club is in good physical enough shape to justify paying a few million.

Let's be honest, if you're going to pay more money for a player than the GDP of a small country it only makes sense that you make damn sure that he's got speed and endurance and is unlikely to pick up an injury due to a pre-existing condition.

Every club will have different medical requirements for new players, but no matter whether the club is Manchester United or Middlesbrough, all checks will be extremely thorough and there'll no way of evading the medical if you are not at the peak of fitness.

Generally, the medical is split into three or four sections, each overseen by a number of different specialists. The first part is invariably undertaken by a team of doctors who carry out a series of measurements, including blood pressure, resting heart rate and an ECG to check that all is in good working order. Some clubs will be especially conscientious in the health of the heart and even conduct an ultrasound scan to ensure the muscle is strong and does not show signs of a condition known as left ventricular hypertrophy.

This condition, although rare, has claimed the lives of a number of world-class footballers over the years and is taken particularly seriously in Italy, where all top athletes are regularly assessed. The doctors hunt for signs that the muscle walls of the left ventricle in the heart are thickening, causing an excessive narrowing in the passageway for the flow of blood. Due to the high intensity of training of footballers and athletes, a degree of thickening is accepted as a normal response. However, in some rare instances, the left ventricle thickens to the point of failure of the heart itself.

Some clubs, as a precaution, insist that part of the medical should involve an ultrasound on the heart and that measurements of the left ventricle chamber be taken to ensure it does not pose a health risk to the player.

The second part of the medical is overseen by an orthopaedic specialist who conducts a very thorough assessment of the player's physical structure – from the health of his knees to the flexibility of his back. These tests can tell the specialists a huge amount about a player and even give clues as to the likelihood of future injuries. For example, if on assessment it is noticed that a player has a pelvic imbalance from a previous injury or a weak core musculature, it could be inferred that he may be predisposed to potential hamstring, groin or back injuries.

In these cases where a player may, at the time of assessment, appear in good working order, yet show signs of potential injury in the future, it would be noted but not necessarily mean he would fail the medical. Of course, if other parts of the medical came back showing he was out of shape, had a slightly dodgy knee and was predisposed to a severe back injury in the near future, the accumulation of 'minor faults' may very well lead to a big cross and no signing.

The third part is the dreaded fitness test. These tests are performed on all players up to three times a season – not just those who are new to the club. In years gone by, the fitness tests which players went through in order to prove their physical worth were pretty raw and involved some very basic fitness testing modalities such as seeing how many shuttle runs a player could perform on a progressively faster sliding scale before collapsing in a heap. These days it is a lot more scientific.

Shuttle runs remain a good all-round way of assessing a player's VO2 max and giving insight into how their mental strength helps them push through the pain barrier. Yet clubs also rely on ready access to high tech laboratory equipment which gives the fitness staff a range of physiological stats to accurately determine the state of their players.

All players are expected to undergo an intense physical assessment of their cardiovascular systems to see how efficient their hearts are at transporting oxygen around the body to the working muscles and how well the body is able to clear lactic acid during intense exercise to enable them to continue running without fatiguing.

Based on these laboratory tests, the fitness team are then incredibly well-positioned to make accurate changes to a player's fitness regime to improve their performance and effectively make their legs more resistant to the effects of accumulating lactic acid.

The main fitness test is performed on a treadmill which starts off slowly and gets progressively quicker throughout the test. In most cases, the initial speed that the player is expected to run is barely faster than a walk but, as the test continues, every minute or so the speed of the treadmill is increased until they are running at near maximum pace.

This test in itself is hard enough but, to make life a little more uncomfortable, for analysis purposes players are wired up to a handful of machines which give a range of information from heart rate to blood pressure, etc. Additionally, they are required to breathe through a special mouthpiece for the duration of the test. The exact levels of oxygen and carbon dioxide inhaled and exhaled can be analysed at the varying intensities they are asked to run at. And, as if that wasn't bad enough, at several stages throughout the test blood samples are taken so that the level of lactic acid in the blood can be analysed. The fitness team assess how much lactic acid is present in the blood and that tells them how well their player can cope with increasing levels in their bloodstream.

All this data is plotted on a series of graphs so the team can see not only if they are in good physical condition but also how they compare to previous testing and if they are in better or worse shape than earlier in the season.

It is likely (although I can't say for sure) that when all results are in from the treadmill test, players will be sat down and their results will be openly discussed and a plan of action decided. If players have demonstrated a drop in fitness levels through nothing more than laziness and a poor commitment to training they will receive the obligatory bollocking, told what level of fitness is expected of them and a programme will then be drawn up for them to follow to reach the required standard. A re-test will then be arranged to make sure they have improved to the satisfaction of the fitness staff.

As the predominant aspect of fitness for a footballer is their cardiovascular ability, it is this aspect which is taken incredibly seriously and dominates a player's fitness training regime. In recent years, thanks to the advances in high-tech fitness assessment equipment, fitness and conditioning coaches have at their disposal some incredibly useful gadgets which help them draw up highly specific cardiovascular training programmes for each player based on their running patterns during a match.

Polar, leaders in heart rate monitoring and fitness assessment, equipment now manufacture special monitoring systems which collate both heart rate and movement data so coaches can tell:

● how far each player runs
● what pace they run at
● how long they run at each pace

With this invaluable data fed back from the sensors, the fitness team can then determine with a great deal of accuracy how far the centre forward or midfielder runs at maximum pace. A training programme can be accurately devised when that information is cross-referenced with heart rate data. This quality of data is priceless for all clubs as it provides highly accurate statistics on each player's running pattern rather than estimating what their level and intensity of training should be.

However, it is not the only aspect of fitness which needs attention.

Current as well as new players will be assessed on their jumping performance, upper body strength and flexibility – an aspect of fitness which is particularly important for goal keepers.

GOAL-KEEPING FITNESS

Keepers are often mocked in training as the running distance they cover in a match isn't exactly far and many question the actual need for keepers to do much fitness training.

Although the distances they run during game might not be the same as that of a midfielder, their level of physical fitness still needs to be exceptional if they are to perform the acrobatic dives which often mean all the difference between winning and losing.

Keepers signing for new clubs undergo an in-depth assessment of their standing jump performance, physical strength and agility which I can guarantee the vast majority of outfield players wouldn't be able to get close to. Hamstrings, hip flexors, back muscles and chest muscles are all assessed to check they have exceptional range of movement so that the body and its limbs are able to move with ease in a split second.

The cardiovascular fitness of keepers is massively underrated by those not in the know. If the heart rate of a keeper is high and they are quickly physically exhausted through not having exceptional anaerobic fitness, they will be unable to perform explosive movements in the air against opposing players and in the mouth of the goal. That means they are effectively no use to the team. In reality, all pro keepers do the same cardiovascular fitness training as their team-mates and they maintain an exceptional level of flexibility.

FITNESS TESTING THE NON-PREMIERSHIP WAY

When it comes to assessing your levels of fitness, due to the (likely) lack of a high-tech treadmill wired up to gaseous exchange, heart rate equipment or an army of sports scientists to tell you what you should be doing, assessing your own fitness levels and knowing how fit you should actually be is very difficult.

All amateur clubs have their own methods of testing players during pre-season, but if you take your game and your fitness levels seriously, you will need to keep tabs on your own fitness levels far more conscientiously than your club does.

The modalities you are going to have to use are a little more basic than those employed by the pros but the tests explained in the following pages are still incredibly effective at giving you a good idea of what your VO2 max is and also monitoring the way in which your fitness levels improve or deteriorate throughout the season.

There are a handful of fitness tests you and a few mates can perform either by yourselves or introduce to be used by your club. All were used until a few years ago in Premiership clubs. Although they are unable to give you the level of information provided in the laboratory, they are still highly effective for you to use at regular intervals throughout the season.

Cooper Test

Like any fitness test, if performed to your maximum potential this one is a real killer.

The protocol of the test is simple – run as far as you can in 12 minutes.

Ideally, a 400-metre running track is the most suitable place to perform this test but seeing that they are not the easiest of training arenas to come across, the most practical place is on a treadmill at your local gym.

All you need to do is set the timer to countdown from 12 mins and play around with the speed until you feel you are running a pace which you can only just about sustain for 12 minutes. This is pretty tricky to judge first time – and potentially dangerous, so be careful and undercook it a little first time you attempt it if necessary. You can always speed up towards the end and try it again another time if you get your pacing wrong.

Once you have tried this test a few times and think you have reached your limit, mark down how many metres you managed to cover and see how you rank using the table below:

Male category	Excellent	Above average	Average	Below average	Poor
20-29	>2800m	2400-2800m	2200-2399m	1600-2199m	<1600m
30-39	>2700m	2300-2700m	1900-2299m	1500-1999m	<1500m
40-49	>2500m	2100-2500m	1700-2099m	1400-1699m	<1400m
>50	>2400m	2000-2400m	1600-1999m	1300-1599m	<1300m

And if you are feeling smug because you are excellent, take a look at how Premiership footballers are ranked based on their results:

Excellent	Above average	Average	Below average	Poor
>3700m	3400-3700m	3100-3399m	2800-3099m	<2800m

If you want to get really serious about this test and obtain a very good estimate on what your VO2 max figure is, simply take the number of metres you ran, subtract 504.9 and divide it by 44.73.

So, for the numerically illiterate (including myself), if you managed to cover 3000 metres the equation would be:

$3000 - 504.9 = 2495.1$

$2495.1 / 44.73 = 55.78$ mls/kg/min

So how would the majority of Premiership footballers fare if they did this test?

Well, if they came in with a VO2 max of 55.78 ml/kg/min

and could only cover 3000 metres in 12 minutes, they would seriously have to reassess their fitness levels and look at improving them. Although an adequate VO2 max level of a player is anywhere from 55 – 65 ml/kg/min, they should really be looking to get into the early 60s at the very least.

CONCLUSION

The Cooper test is very easy to perform, requiring little equipment other than a 400m running track or a treadmill – and most people will have access to the latter. It certainly gives you a good idea of how fit you are, but the one minor drawback is that it is not really very specific for football. Sure, it lets you know how far you can run over 12 minutes, but when was the last time you ran at any pace for longer than 12 seconds on the football field? The game is played in a stop-start manner, brief periods of intense exercise followed by a gentle jog, so although useful to integrate into a fitness testing programme, the Cooper test is not sufficiently football-specific to be relied upon as a sole measure of cardiovascular fitness.

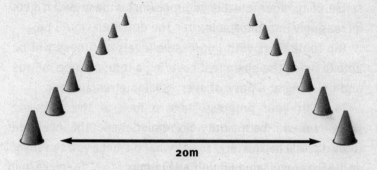

20m

THE BLEEP TEST

The bleep test has been the staple form of testing the fitness of footballers and rugby players for years. It is an excellent technique and was used extensively by the top clubs until technology took over and training took a more scientific approach.

The bleep or 'multi-stage fitness' test is challenging and can predict your VO2 max and highlight any shortfalls in your cardiovascular conditioning.

The test is performed between two 20-metre markers between which the participant runs continuously. These shuttle runs are synchronised with a pre-recorded CD or MP3, which plays a series of bleeps at set intervals. The interval between each successive beep gets progressively shorter, forcing the runner to increase speed until they are unable to keep up.

The test starts with the beeps so far apart that you can pretty much walk between the markers – but don't let the easy start fool you. As time goes on, those beeps get closer and closer together and gradually you will start to lose your sense of humour and begin running at a pace which gets increasingly uncomfortable.

Top footballers with impressive levels of fitness will be able to finish the bleep test covering a total of 4900 metres and finishing at a pace of over 18 kilometres an hour.

To chart your progress, take a look at the following table taken from the Sports Coach UK website (www.sportscoachuk.org) to see what distance you can cover and what speed you end up finishing on.

Levels	Shuttles	Kilometres per hour	Seconds per shuttle	Total level time in seconds	Distance in metres	Total distance	Total time
1	7	8.0	9.0	63.0	140	140	1.03
2	8	9.0	8.0	64.0	160	300	2.07
3	8	9.5	7.58	60.63	160	460	3.08
4	9	10.0	7.20	64.80	180	640	4.12
5	9	10.5	6.86	61.71	180	820	5.14
6	9	11.0	6.55	58.91	180	1000	6.13
7	10	11.5	6.26	62.61	200	1200	7.16
8	10	12.0	6.0	60.0	200	1400	8.16
9	11	12.5	5.76	63.36	220	1620	9.19
10	11	13.0	5.54	60.92	220	1840	10.20
11	12	13.5	5.33	64.0	240	2080	11.24
12	12	14.0	5.14	61.71	240	2320	12.26
13	13	14.5	4.97	64.55	260	2580	13.30
14	13	15.0	4.80	62.40	260	2840	14.33
15	13	15.5	4.65	60.39	260	3100	15.33
16	14	16.0	4.50	63.0	280	3380	16.36
17	14	16.5	4.36	61.09	280	3660	17.37
18	15	17.0	4.24	63.53	300	3960	18.41
19	15	17.5	4.11	61.71	300	4260	19.42
20	16	18.0	4.00	64.0	320	4580	20.46
21	16	18.5	3.89	62.27	320	4900	21.49

The multi-stage fitness test incurs a total distance of 4900 metres in a time of 21.49.

© The National Coaching Foundation, 2008

The great thing about this test is that any number of people can perform it at the same time, provided they are near enough to hear the bleep and by competing against team-mates it makes the test that much more competitive and drives players to the limits of physical exhaustion.

This test should ideally be performed at the beginning of the season and used to give you an idea on how fit you are currently – and a target to try and beat next time.

To give you an idea on your estimated VO2 max, take a look at the following VO2 max estimations based on the level you finish on:

Level 7 =	36.6 ml/kg/min
Level 8 =	40 ml/kg/min
Level 9 =	43.4 ml/kg/min
Level 10 =	46.9 ml/kg/min
Level 11 =	50.2 ml/kg/min
Level 12=	53.8 ml/kg/min
Level 13=	57.3 ml/kg/min

CONCLUSION

Although the bleep test has now fallen out of favour with the top clubs, it still remains a fantastic fitness test for amateur footballers throughout the season to keep track of fitness levels. It is not the ultimate test, as some players may have a low VO2 max, but are able to function at a high percentage of their maximum capacity for long periods of time but, all in all, it is the one test which most fitness coaches would suggest you use to monitor your cardiovascular capacity.

However, like the Cooper tests, the continuous nature of the shuttle runs does not accurately replicate the stop-start nature of the game. This is where the yo-yo test comes in.

THE YO-YO TEST

Of all the fitness tests you can do outside of the laboratory, the yo-yo is arguably one of the best tests of cardiovascular fitness you can do and it is highly specific to the requirements of football.

Like both the Cooper and bleep tests, the principle is easy, but practice is very hard.

There are several versions of the test, each one designed for use with differing levels of fitness.

Endurance and intermittent yo-yo tests are similar to the bleep. The one key difference is in the intermittent version, when players can take a brief rest between shuttle runs. This brief rest period makes the test much more like the sort of conditions under which you'd play a real game of football and is therefore a far more accurate way of assessing player fitness.

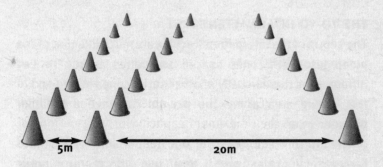

THE YO-YO ENDURANCE TEST

The yo-yo endurance test is a continuous variation of the bleep. A version of the test is designed for beginners (level one) and a separate one is for advanced athletes (level two). The level one test is effectively the same as the standard bleep test described earlier and is suitable for recreational footballers. Advance to level two and it becomes a very difficult game. The test starts at a higher running speed and has bigger increments in speed – making life pretty miserable early on, as you struggle to keep pace with the relentless beeps which get forever closer together.

It goes without saying that Premiership players are no longer expected to perform these tests very often, if at all, due to the more intricate assessment methods that their teams now use in the lab. That said, if the conditioning coach wants to teach a player a lesson then they would certainly get them to perform the level two yo-yo test. Depending on the player's indiscretion, however, there is every chance they would also be expected to take on the intermittent yo-yo test.

THE YO-YO INTERMITTENT TEST

The set up of the intermittent test is very much like that of the bleep test, with cones spaced 20 metres apart. The key difference is there usually another set of cones at one end of the testing area where the players can take a breather between intervals.

The intermittent version is also divided into level one for recreational players and a level two with faster running speeds and bleeps aimed at the professional player.

The protocol is simply to run to the end cone and back again, keeping time with beeps. At the end of each shuttle run, the participant will take a ten-second break before the shuttle has to be performed again. As the test goes on, the bleeps get closer and closer together and the test concludes when the player stops (or more likely collapses in a heap on the floor, gasping for air and shedding a few tears).

Like any test, it important that the level you reach before you can no longer continue is recorded so that you can chart future fitness improvements against your previous test. In the yo- yo test, you should record the total distance covered before you can no longer keep up with the bleeps.

The following table is a summary of the total distance you are likely to cover while doing the level one intermittent test, as this is the one which is likely to be best-suited to your fitness ability:

Level	Speed	Shuttles of 2 x 20 metres	Accumulated distance covered in metres
1	10	1	40
2	11.5	1	80
3	13	2	160
4	13.5	3	280
5	14	4	440
6	14.5	8	760
7	15	8	1080
8	15.5	8	1400
9	16	8	1720
10	16.5	8	2040
11	17	8	2360
12	17.5	8	2680
13	18	8	3000
14	18.5	8	3320
15	19	8	3640

Table taken from www.topendsports.com

This test, as with all others, is not for the faint-hearted, so before you decide to push yourself with any of these high-intensity assessments, make sure you have a good level of fitness and no pre-existing health conditions.

According to a leading Premiership strength and conditioning coach, the pick of the bunch is the yo-yo test. It is one which most accurately replicates fitness required for football and, with the help of very affordable heart-rate monitoring equipment, the test can be made even more effective.

HEART RATE MONITORING FOR SUPREME FITNESS GAINS

It doesn't have to be the intermittent yo-yo. Any test is fantastic for keeping tabs on your fitness levels during the season. All you need to do is a quick Cooper, bleep or yo-yo every couple of months or so and compare your result against your last effort. Assuming you have trained properly and put the hard work in to improve your cardiovascular efficiency, you should notice some pretty significant performance improvements in terms of being able to run further before fatiguing and collapsing in a heap.

However, you're really missing a trick if the sole method you are using to chart fitness gains is simply trying to run a bit further than the last time you tested yourself. Don't get me wrong – relying on this method is a great gauge and far better than not performing fitness tests at all, but by using a heart rate monitor for fitness testing and training, you can gather so much more information about your fitness levels and put yourself in a far more informed position for tweaking your training programme to ensure maximum fitness gains. By using a heart rate monitor in conjunction with the fitness tests you can compare your heart rate at any given stage of the test with previous results. Regularly check your heart rate before, during and after training and gain a physiological insight into how your heart responds to training. You will be able to confirm that it is getting stronger and more efficient at supplying the muscles with the oxygen they need to function at maximal capacity.

THE TOP HEART-RATE TRAINING MYTHS

Whenever I am asked by keen footballers and runners about the best way to improve aerobic capacity and fitness levels, the first thing I ask is – do they use a heart rate monitor? The response is usually:

- A heart what?
- I'm not a professional, so why do I need one?
- I thought about it but don't you need a degree in sports science to work out target training zones?
- Aren't they really expensive?

It's true to say that the benefits of training with a heart rate monitor are better known to the general sporting public than they were a decade ago, but there is still a belief that the equipment is inaccessible – too expensive or too complicated to integrate into a training regime. This is simply not the case.

Firstly, the aptly-named www.heartratemonitor.co.uk sells a huge selection of devices with prices from as little as £30 to models costing over £300 for the seriously gadget-minded. But you don't need the most expensive version. Ask any personal trainer or Premiership fitness coach and they will tell you that spending £30 on a heart rate monitor is the best investment you can make in improving your fitness levels – bar none.

Secondly, although I agree that the science behind heart rate training can be pretty complicated, there are certain principles which are easy to understand and which I will outline in the following pages. By all means, feel free to read an in-depth book on heart rate training if you are interested in using it to its maximum effect, but the tips explained in this section of the book cover all the basic information you need to use a heart rate monitor with your training.

WHY USE A HEART RATE MONITOR?

Premiership conditioning coaches have used heart rate monitors on their players for years. The first team monitoring system was manufactured by Polar in 2000 when the technology was still expensive. It was then an inaccessible luxury for anyone but the professionals and it was way out of reach of the average lower-division player. This has now all changed and the benefits of heart rate training are well worth the vastly reduced outlay required these days to acquire one.

Despite the fact that your thigh muscles are responsible for winning matches through being the powerhouse which drive the ball into the net, it is actually your heart muscle that gets you around the park in the first place. Your thighs may very well win you adoring looks from hundreds of potential

WAGS on the sidelines but it is your heart which needs to be trained to be able to tolerate the demands of an intense 90-minute game of football.

Your heart is the pump responsible for supplying essential, nutrient-rich blood to your thighs and if it is not up to the job and too weak to work hard enough to supply demand then – no matter how sculpted your legs are – they won't have a decent supply of oxygenated blood to power them and you'll be useless to your team-mates. By training your heart scientifically with a heart rate monitor, you'll be able to accurately train within certain targets for specific periods of time, making the quality of your training far better.

Premiership players spend virtually the whole of pre-season wearing a heart rate monitor so that conditioning staff can tell exactly how hard their hearts are working at any given intensity. If it is noted that a certain player is working too hard at certain intensities and he shouldn't be finding the training as tough as his readout indicates, then the fitness team know that more work needs to be done to make sure that player's heart is strengthened and better able to tolerate the intensity.

Although the systems used by the Premiership are way outside your budget, a modestly-priced monitor can give you one hell of a lot of information and feedback on your pre-season training and it's worth its weight in gold. The top teams provide each player with a uniquely-coded heart rate strap and a speed sensor. The fitness team sit on the sidelines with a laptop on which they gather heart rate and speed information from every player – in real time.

The benefits of this are massive, as heart rate and running speeds can be compared directly to those achieved in previous training drills and the conditioning staff can tell when their players' fitness levels are improving, when they stay the same or – worst case scenario – showing a decrease. Whatever their individual heart rate stats, every player can be individually assessed and their personal training regimes can be easily tweaked to ensure they meet expected standards of fitness by the beginning of the season. Without heart rate monitors, the accuracy of their training programmes would be based on guesswork and it's not difficult to see why Polar report that 95 per cent of Premiership teams and 76 per cent of all major league teams use heart rate monitors to assess players.

And the best bit is that your cheaper monitor will be able to give you virtually all the information you need and will last you for years. The only thing you need to know is how to use it.

MEASURING YOUR HEART RATE AT REST

Once you have your monitor, and worked out how to turn it on and get a heart rate reading, the next obvious step is to find out how to use it to improve your fitness levels. The novelty of staring down at the watch receiver watching your heart rate jump from around 60-70 beats a minute to 80-90 beats a minute when you visualise a passionate encounter with Angelina Jolie and then drop again when you picture Nora Batty are fun for a bit, but at some time or other you're going to have to get training.

You can start off by taking a reading of your true 'resting heart rate' (RHR). Although the reasons for getting a particular result vary from person to person, generally speaking the lower your heart rate is at rest, the larger your heart muscle and the fitter you are. By regularly testing your resting heart rate you can gauge if you are effectively training your heart properly and making it stronger.

Due to natural (and unnatural) fluctuations in resting heart rate, it is important to be consistent when you take a reading. The best time to take a RHR reading is first thing in the morning, as soon as you wake up. Not only does this make repeat readings more accurate being taken at the same time of day, but there are fewer external factors to lead to a false reading.

The easiest way to take it is to strap on your heart rate monitor, lie down and measure your heart rate for about five minutes. Most models costing somewhere in the region of £50 have an average heart rate function, making it easy to take a reading over five minutes which you'll then be able log in a diary for future comparison.

If you do not have a heart monitor, simply find the point of your strongest pulse –usually on your wrist (in the radial artery) or under your jaw (the carotid artery). Use a regular watch or timer to count the number of beats you feel in 30 seconds and then double it. You have the figure for your RHR.

Make a point of recording your RHR once a week over the course of your training. Provided you are putting the work in and training hard within your suggested heart rate limits (these will be explained later), you will begin to notice a gradual decrease in resting heart rate. This proves that your heart muscle is getting stronger and fitness levels are improving. The stronger your heart gets the more blood it is able to eject with every beat, which is why your resting heart rate will drop. Your heart simply does not have to work as hard to provide the muscles and your body with the oxygen and nutrients it needs to survive. The hearts of top players often get as low as 40 beats a minute, but as a mortal with less time available to train you can probably expect your resting heart rate to drop from 60 beats a minute to around 50 beats a minute.

Don't be surprised if every now and again your resting heart rate gives you a reading which is either higher or lower than you'd expect. There are a number of reasons why – despite training yourself into the ground for two weeks – your resting heart rate can give you a higher reading that you'd expect.

For example, the hormone adrenaline has a direct effect on your heart and can increase its rate enormously – which is why you see frenzied medical staff in hospital dramas ram a massive syringe full of adrenaline directly into a patient whose heart has stopped beating.

Most of the time you don't have direct control over the amount of adrenaline your body produces (if you're interested, it's secreted in the adrenal medulla near the liver). Increased adrenaline levels are often a response of our fight-or-flight instinct and occur when we are frightened or even emotionally revved up before a big match.

The main causes of an increased rate of adrenaline into our blood stream are:

● Caffeine intake
● Anticipation of exercise or an upcoming occasion/event
● Stress

Caffeine stimulates the adrenal glands to secrete an increased quantity of adrenaline, especially in those who do not consume it regularly. As a result, a harmless cup of coffee half an hour before a RHR test can produce an elevated reading, though the same effect from coffee can actually play to your advantage as a way to enhance your physical performance on the field – more about this will be explained in chapter 5.

The anticipation of exercise or an important upcoming event is often understated but highly influential on the heart at rest. I have witnessed a client's heart rate rise from 100 beats a minute to 150 beats a minute in around three minutes by sitting still and focusing on performing an intense 500 metre-sprint on a rowing machine.

Increased stress levels from family problems or work related issues can also cause an elevated level of adrenaline in the bloodstream. It causes the heart to beat higher at rest than it should. This happens to all of us once in a while, but if you feel you have been stressed for a while and you are training hard to improve your fitness levels for the upcoming season it is advisable to have regular medical check-ups just to make sure you heart is not unduly affected by the emotional and physical battering it is getting at the same time. Adrenaline is good – but too much of it can be a serious health problem.

Resting heart rate can be a little higher than you expected if you have an oncoming cold or illness. In fact, unexplained increases in resting heart rate can be an excellent way of foreseeing poor health.. Experienced Premiership players who regularly keep tabs on their RHR can often tell if they will come down with a cold in a few days by simply noticing an increase of around ten beats a minute in resting and exercising heart rate.

So if you have been putting some serious training in (which can in fact compromise your immune system for a short period of time) and you are finding your heart rate is higher than you'd expect both at rest and during exercise, there is a strong possibility you will be reaching for the tissues in a couple of days.

Environmental temperature can affect your heart at rest as well as during exercise. When the body is exposed to a temperature it is unused to, blood is diverted closer to the skin where it can cool down, resulting in an increased heart rate. So when you note down your resting heart rate, it's a good idea to also make a note of the ambient temperature. You don't necessarily have to know the exact temperature, but 'cold', 'average' or 'hot' is certainly worth recording to keep your readings consistent.

All tests should be performed at the same temperature every time – irrespective of the time of the year. This is one of the reasons why Premiership fitness testing has now moved indoors, away from performing tests such as the yo-yo test on the pitch where climatic conditions can vary hugely. In the lab climate control keeps the temperature constant and testing far more accurate.

You can delve deeper into the reasons why your resting heart rate can give you rogue results despite hard training. There are dozens more reasons for an increased RHR and some may require medical intervention. Elevated blood calcium levels and increased thyroid hormone secretion are two examples which require medical treatment. It is also worth noting that certain medications can be responsible for artificially raising heart rate, a situation worth discussing with your physician.

REASONS FOR LOW RHR

People with a low RHR often suffer from low blood pressure. Though not necessarily a problem, short-lived symptoms of dizziness and light headiness can occur when standing up quickly from a lying or seated position. It can become a bit of an annoyance – especially when people automatically assume you've been drinking.

Generally speaking, there are fewer common reasons for a RHR to be abnormally low. Although increasing your fitness levels will significantly lower your rate, this is certainly not detrimental to your health. Medication also strongly influences cardiac response. Beta blockers or pills for hypertension (high blood pressure) can be a cause of low heart rate, so take extra care if you are on such medication.

Also see a doctor if you have a prolonged period of low resting heart rate with symptoms of lethargy and fatigue. These can be an indication of hypothyroidism and can go for on for months without diagnosis. If your training is harder than you think and you feel under the weather, it is certainly worth getting yourself looked at.

MEASURING YOUR HEART RATE DURING EXERCISE

Although measuring your resting heart rate should be an integral part of your training regime, it is far more important to know what your training heart rate should be – so that you can make those fitness gains in the first place.

Although it is certainly a myth that you need a degree in sports science to effectively set yourself heart-rate training zones, it is still pretty tricky to come up with a series of accurate training zones to suit everyone.

Due to variance in our builds, muscularity, fitness levels and cardiac physiology it would be impossible for me to provide one hundred per cent accurate zones for you to train in. I can give you the tools to work it out yourself based on your ability as an athlete, but ultimately you are the one who will have to tweak your training in order to really make the heart rate monitor work for you and make an impact on your training levels.

SO WHERE DO YOU START?

The best place to start is to find out your maximum possible heart rate – also known, unsurprisingly, as your heart rate max (HR max). Once you know how many times your heart is able to beat in one minute, you are then able to create for yourself some very accurate heart rate zones, in which you must work in, in order to make your training football specific.

The best way to accurately discover your true maximum heart rate is not really much fun but if you have a fitness coach who just loves beasting you in pre-season, it's a great idea to strap on your heart rate monitor for the duration of the session and take a glance at the monitor when you collapse in a mess on the floor, as this is likely to be the point where you have reached your HR max.

To accurately find out the true maximum number of times your heart will beat in a minute, exercise to complete exhaustion – a process which not only taxes you physically but requires mental strength. It sorts the men from the boys and only you know if you're man enough to handle it. Do remember that exercising to exhaustion can be very stressful to the body if you are not used to high-intensity work, so only follow this protocol if you are already reasonably well-conditioned.

While you are tested in the training park under the watchful eye of your sadistic fitness coach, most Premiership players have their maximum heart rate assessed in a controlled environment. The tests are usually performed on a treadmill, but can be done on an exercise bike or rowing machine. Regardless of which modality is used, the chances are that the test will not be complete until you have pushed your body to its physical limits and can no longer sustain exercise.

Fortunately for the girls among you who are scared of pain there is an easier way to find out your maximal heart rate without subjecting yourself to what feels like a near death experience. However, this method is not particularly accurate and can affect your calculations when working out your training zones. To find out your *theoretical* maximum heart rate all you need to do is simply subtract your age from 220.

For example:

If you are 30 years old, it's 220 – 30 = 190.

Therefore, theoretically, the maximum number of times your heart can beat in one minute is 190 times.

Unfortunately, as with many principles in this book, individuality plays a significant role in making this theory potentially useless. This formula is very useful as a guide, but in reality I have found very few people who find it accurate.

Many players, especially those of 'mature' years, are able to run quite happily with a rate well above their theoretical maximum. In fact according to leading sports physiologists David Costill and Jack Wilmore, 68 per cent of 40-year-olds have an actual maximum heart rate of between 168 and 192 beats per minute. And 95 per cent of 40-year-olds have a maximum heart rate which falls in the range of 156-192 beats per minute.

As a general rule, the younger you are the more likely this formula will apply to you – but don't count on it. If you notice during a hard training session that your heart rate exceeds your theoretical maximum, adjust it accordingly and make a note of the highest rate that you recorded and use that figure as your HR max.

Once you have a pretty good idea what your maximum heart rate is, the next step to ensuring you get maximum fitness gains is to work out how many beats per minute your heart should be pumping during certain training drills. There is no point in investing in a heart monitor if you don't know how hard your heart should be working at any given training intensity. Use the following information to your advantage and train smarter – not necessarily harder.

Your heart rate is basically a measurement of the demand placed on your cardio-respiratory system during training when it has to deliver sufficient levels of oxygen to working muscles so that exercise intensity can be maintained. Over time, as a result of your training, your heart will adapt to the stresses being asked of it, making it more efficient. The workload you once found tough will become a breeze.

To illustrate this point, take a look at the graph below to get a visual idea of what happens to your heart rate when you train properly and your fitness levels increase. By following the correct training protocols, your heart will respond to training as shown in the graph. Not only will it not need to work nearly as hard at a given workload but you will also be able to run faster and further than you could before training.

Of course, provided you do the actual training these physiological adaptations would take place whether you use a heart rate monitor or not, but the advantage of using one is that you can not only tell during your training that you are

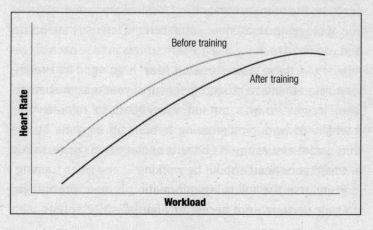

running at the right intensity but you can also tell categorically that your heart has got stronger and more efficient by noticing a similar trend in your heart rate data as in the graph above.

WHAT PERCENTAGE OF HR MAX SHOULD YOU WORK AT?

So what percentage will get you match-fit and super-charged for the season?

Running at a variety of percentages of your maximum heart rate for certain lengths of time is essential to get your body to adapt to the physical demands of a football match. However, generally speaking, the higher percentage you train at the better.

One mistake some players make every year is to embark on long training runs at a modest 70-75 per cent of their maximum heart rate and wonder why they are blowing out of their ass in the first game of the season. It shouldn't be a surprise: the running demands of football are varied; at times you are jogging along slowly and then the intensity shoots up and you need to make five 30-yard sprints in the space of two minutes. In these instances your heart is going to be beating far quicker than at a poxy 70 per cent of your maximum heart rate. If you haven't trained your heart to tolerate this intensity of work, you're going to slow up big time by the third sprint and you won't be able to make that crucial tackle or the vital clearance kick.

Premiership players spend a lot of their pre-season training performing a series of high intensity sprints with gradually reduced recovery times. They train their hearts to adapt to performing at high rates and are still able to maintain a fast running pace.

HOW DO THEY DO IT?

The secret is to work out a training timetable of say six weeks and gradually increase the intensity of training over time.

By the end of the training programme, you notice:

- Your heart rate will be lower than it was at the same intensity at the beginning of training
- Your heart will recover far quicker in your rest periods between interval runs, making it easier for you to perform the next interval at the correct intensity
- You will be able to tolerate training at high heart rates as your body becomes more efficient at clearing away lactic acid from the muscles – meaning you can continue training without feeling exhausted

ANAEROBIC HEART-RATE TRAINING AND THE SECRET OF GETTING MATCH FIT

I've made it clear that heading out for a five-mile jog at 75 per cent of your maximum heart rate is not the best way to maximise your fitness gains for the duration of your pre-season training. By all means, include a steady jog once a week in your training programme, but do not let low intensity training dominate your training timetable.

You should be aiming to be training hard enough to require more than oxygen to fuel movement. This is anaerobic training – at a heart rate of 85 per cent or more. This will ensure you build up a tolerance to the high intensity running demanded by the game of football.

Your training should include a series of sprints at 85 per cent of your maximum pace for 30 seconds (early in pre-season) to sprints at one hundred per cent, for 5-10 seconds (performed toward the end). You'll be well above the 85 per cent mark overall and that will give your heart and your legs the strength they need to tolerate the physiological demands of short, sharp sprints.

Everyone trains differently and each coach will have their own approach for getting you match fit, but you use the following sample training programme to give you an idea about how to best use your heart rate monitor to improve fitness levels. You'll need to record your heart rate data after every interval, so it would make life easier if you had a heart rate monitor with a 'lap' or interval function on it. This will automatically record data for you.

In the following sample training programme (which is pretty tame) you should see your heart rate reach above 80 per cent of its max for the majority of the training session. If it doesn't – run faster!

WARM-UP
Always have a good ten-minute warm-up prior to each session. Jog around the paddock a few times dribbling the ball, getting progressively faster – and remember to stretch.

Repeat each session three times over the week.

WEEK ONE

● Perform 5-8 fast runs at 80 per cent of your maximum speed (not heart rate). Run from the goal up to the halfway line and back. Rest for 30 seconds

● *Record your heart rate at the end and beginning of each interval*

● Rest for three minutes. Repeat the exercise, recording your heart rate at the end and beginning of each interval

WEEK TWO

● Perform 5-8 fast runs at 80 per cent of your maximum speed (not heart rate). Run from the goal up to the halfway line and back. Rest for 25 seconds

● *Record your heart rate at the end and beginning of each interval*

● Rest for two minutes. Repeat the whole session twice (not forgetting to record your heart rate each time)

WEEK THREE

● Perform 8-12 fast runs at 80-85 per cent of your maximum speed (not heart rate). Run from the goal up to the halfway line and back. Rest for 20 seconds

● *Record your heart rate at the end and beginning of each interval*

● Have a two-minute break. Repeat the session twice more, recording heart rate data each time

When you've finished the programme, go back and do the exercises from the first week. Note the data as before and compare your heart rate to those initial readings. You should see massive drops in heart rate both immediately after your interval and in your rate of recovery. It's also highly likely that you will have run faster – and at a lower heart rate.

This will give you confidence that your training is paying off and you will be able to see the physiological benefits of performing high intensity training runs. It will also serve as a good indicator of where your fitness levels are throughout the season.

For example, perform the week one training session following a four-week lay-off from injury and see how your rate compares. This will give you a good idea of how much fitness you have lost and how hard you need to work to get it back.

To get the most out of your season you have to keep tabs on your fitness levels. Premiership players may have every specialist under the sun to help them maximise their time training but the tips and tools explained in this chapter are excellent resources to help you train that much more precisely.

Using techniques and principles such as heart-rate training and yo-yo tests, your pre-season training should be far more productive than any you've previously experienced. The key thing now is to make sure every training session you do from the first day of pre-season to the last is at the right intensities and for the right times to maximise your fitness gains.

CHAPTER THREE
PRE-SEASON
TRAINING
PHYSICAL FINE TUNING

Back in 1979, just months after Geoff Hurst took the reins as manager of Chelsea, he gave the players a little surprise. A surprise that would have had some players licking their lips with excitement while instilling in others an insatiable desire to fake injury and go home. Hurst had recruited loyal Chelsea fan and Olympic champion Sebastian Coe to show the players what high-intensity anaerobic fitness was really all about.

Left-winger Clive Walker admitted quite openly that Coe brought a new meaning to the word 'fitness'. His sessions involved a series of football-specific training drills, including the all-important 60-yard sprint. However, as Walker points out, 'We would do ten runs of 60-yards each and he [Coe] would do double that amount with ease.

Okay, so Sebastian Coe's ball control and vision of space

was probably far from Premiership standard, but his superior level of anaerobic fitness certainly gave the Chelsea's 'class of '79' something to think about.

Even if you've got all the ball skills in the world, you won't be a class player unless your anaerobic fitness is awesome. You need to aim for the physical ability to run at pace *and* at a high percentage of your maximum heart rate for long periods *and* develop the ability to recover quickly and do it all over again over the course of 90 minutes. Only then can you truly get the most out of yourself as a top-class player.

Vision, awareness of space, guile and fancy footwork are essential but conditioning your body to perform dozens of fast anaerobic runs over the course of a 90-minute match is crucial – and pre-season is the ideal time to do just that.

To a degree just how fit you get in time for the start of the season is up to you as an amateur or recreational player. Sure, your club coach will shout and scream at you for a couple of weeks and will get you to do shuttle runs, etc, but if you are really serious about getting into good anaerobic shape you are going to have to do a lot more outside those twice-weekly sessions.

Interestingly, it might surprise you to learn that this doesn't just apply to lower league players. The same thing is true at the top of the Premiership tree.

You might justifiably assume that the best players need only turn up for their pre-season fitness training sessions, do what is asked of them and then go home and (pay someone to) polish their Bentley. In many cases this is not true. A leading Premiership fitness coach told me that players are advised to work on their core musculature and upper body strength outside their individually-tailored training sessions. I asked how this was 'policed' and was actually quite shocked to hear him say: 'It isn't. We can't mollycoddle the players and be like a headmaster. They are all adults and we feel they should be given the responsibility to train on their own – for their own good.'

'And do they?' I asked.

'Some do, some don't,' he told me. 'Some players are obsessed with their levels of fitness and are always asking what their VO2 max is and whether they are fitter than they were six weeks ago. They'll spend much of their spare time in the gym working hard on their fitness levels to make them the best players they can be. On the other hand, sadly, there are others who will do the bare minimum asked of them and need a lot of coercing to get their asses into the gym them. Sadly, although they are in the minority and often the younger ones, some players are just happy to pick up their weekly pay cheque and do just enough to get through the 90 minutes.'

Despite having all the resources available to them, there are some highly prominent footballers – who I cannot name – who are a little complacent when it comes to their fitness and rely on their skill levels more than their fitness to justify their weekly wage.

Great if you can get away with it, but not one fitness coach or league manager would recommend you take this attitude to the game. Physical fitness drills and body conditioning during pre-season is key to your team's ultimate success at the end of the season, so take it seriously but above all – do it properly.

STRETCHING

As explained in Chapter 1, the importance of stretching and improving a player's flexibility is grossly underrated – at all levels of the game. You'd be amazed at how poor the flexibility of some of the Premiership footballers is. They invite injury after injury until they sort it out.

Stretching is important throughout the season – both on and off the pitch – but pre-season is when fitness coaches read the riot act to players about the importance of doing it regularly – and how to go about it properly.

Players at the top level now know how to stretch correctly thanks to specialists taking them through a series of key stretches which help to safely elongate their muscle fibres without risking injury and others which help to 'wake up' the nervous system and get their body physiologically prepared for training or playing.

Unless you are well clued-up about the science behind performance-enhancing stretching, it's likely your stretching routine will be very different to the one John Terry and co go through before every game – but now you're going to have a chance to emulate their routines.

While several Premiership fitness coaches were helpful with various aspects of this book, they were all equally unwilling to give away in-depth information on how they get the player's muscles stretched before a game. This level of secrecy is in itself fascinating, an indication of just how important the pros themselves view the art of stretching. They simply wouldn't dare to reveal anything for me. And when I pushed them, they all told me bluntly the same thing. They didn't know what stretching, testing or fitness routines were used by rival clubs – so why on earth would they confide their own secrets?

Fair enough.

However, having taken a few educational trips to the USA and by calling upon my own extensive experience in the fitness industry, I am able to give you very good idea about top stretching protocols. Some are vital, some are largely banned due to risk of injury and some are stretches you can do before a game which will ensure you are full of life and ready to take on the full 90-minutes as soon as the whistle goes.

It is essential that you warm up the muscles before performing any stretch. The start of any training session or match warm up should include at least 5-10 minutes of gentle jogging to encourage blood flow to the muscles and make them more pliable and receptive to stretching. Failure to do so could easily result in a muscle tear, so always go for a good jog around the pitch a few times before you even consider stretching out those hammies.

STATIC STRETCHING

Static stretching is perhaps one of the most common types of stretching seen up and down the country, both in gyms and on the football pitch.

As the name suggests, static stretching is performed with

the muscle placed at the point of stretch and held. The duration of the stretch is between 10-15 seconds. Classic examples include grabbing hold of one foot and pulling it towards your bum to stretch your thighs and extending one leg and leaning towards it to stretch your hamstrings.

These stretches are best to do progressively, either at the beginning of your warm-up regime – as one of the first stretches you do after a light jog – or at home after exercising to help improve flexibility over a period of time. They're not so great before a game. The static nature of this stretch help to elongate the muscle fibres and put them in a better state to contract but, neurologically, the stretch is poor preparation for the match. Holding the muscle still does nothing to wake the nerves in your legs when you want to get them excited about the prospect of exercise.

Many players fall into this trap and spend a good deal of time statically stretching their quads and hamstrings before kick-off. The result is that you start the game feeling sluggish and far from being up for it. Static stretching definitely has its place in helping to improve flexibility but use it sparingly in the moments leading up to the start of the game.

BALLISTIC STRETCHING

A very old school style of stretching, ballistic or bounce stretching was the norm a few years ago and thought to be a great way to warm up the hamstrings. But stretch is responsible for high instances of muscle tweaks and most (experienced and knowledgeable coaches) have now all but consigned it to Room 101.

The classic ballistic stretch involves standing with the legs either together or apart and leaning forwards, with the arms hanging towards the floor. The stretch is then performed by lowering your hands as toward the ground as far as your hamstrings will allow and then bounce back up again a few centimetres and then reach for the ground again. This stretch is then repeated over and over again until eventually your hands are able to touch the ground.

It might be an effective stretch and you may very well see your hamstring flexibility improve by a good six inches but the risk is not worth the potential rewards. And that risk? You are never fully in control. Your whole upper body weight is essentially being forced upon your hamstring muscles (and if your legs are wide apart it will also be taken by the adductor muscles). You are not in an easy position to pull out of the stretch or reduce its intensity if your hamstrings are not sufficiently warm.

It is because of this lack of control that ballistic stretching is best avoided – if you value the health of your hamstrings. You might get away with it 99 times out of 100 but if you are one of those people who are naturally tight (in the muscle sense) that one time may tweak a hamstring and leave you on the sidelines for a few weeks.

DYNAMIC STRETCHING

Now we're talking proper performance enhancing stretching.

Dynamic stretching is arguably the best way to get your muscles and entire body physiologically ready for a game. All Premiership players will do long periods of dynamic stretching for all major muscles in the build-up to the game and there is no reason why you can't do the same.

Up until fairly recently, the benefits of dynamic stretching were not well understood, especially in lower division clubs where if any stretching at all was to take place it would be static. Now the word has got out and the use of dynamic stretching is widespread, though I am sometimes surprised to see good players still rely on the old school versions.

Put simply, a dynamic stretch is one which involves moving areas of your body such as your legs, gradually increasing the range and speed of movement over a period of time.

Always go on a 5-10 minute jog before dynamic stretching in order to encourage a decent amount of blood flow to the leg muscles. By all means follow that run with a series of static stretches if you wish, but overall the pre-match warm-up should finish with dynamic stretches.

Take your hamstrings as examples. To dynamically stretch those all-important (and injury-prone) hammies, stand up straight and hold onto a team-mate or an immoveable object such as the goal post. This isn't essential, but it does make it that much easier to perform the stretch without falling over and looking like an idiot. Slowly start to swing one of your legs in front of you in a pendulum motion and gradually increase the range of the swing over a 30-second period. Over the course of that time you'll find that the stretch will get progressively easier as the hamstring muscle fibres gradually stretch and become accustomed to the increased range of motion you are putting them through. After a few seconds swap legs and repeat with the other one.

To get maximum benefit from this stretch and to really wake up the nerves, repeat this stretch three or four times and gradually increase the speed at which you swing your leg. The combination of the increased range of motion and the speed at which your hamstring muscle fibres stretch will significantly impact your nervous system and nicely fire up your legs for kick off.

You can wear a heart rate monitor while performing this stretch. Take a look at what happens to your heart rate during the stretch and notice how much it increases. This in itself should make it clear just how good dynamic stretching is in the build-up to the game.

Static stretching barely budges the heart rate above 100 beats per minute and it's not difficult to work out which style you should be spending most of your time doing in the 30 minutes before a game.

Of course, dynamic stretching can be applied generally. It's not just the hamstrings. All muscles can be stretched gradually by increasing their range and speed of movement. Your thighs, for example, can be dynamically stretched by jogging along and kicking your heels towards your butt. Gradually increase the speed that you exercise to improve the stretch.

Your adductors too can be dynamically stretched. Good old side steps are fantastic for warming up the insides of your legs and preparing them for battle. As you exercise, gradually increase the width and speed of the steps.

Always remember to warm up the muscles first. When you do dynamic stretches – as opposed to ballistic stretching – you are always in full control of the range of motion you put your muscles through, but you must make them pliable and in the right state to be worked on. The only way to do this is to make sure they are warm by going for a light jog first. Always start the stretch gently and progressively increase the range of motion.

BREAKING IT ALL DOWN WITH PRE-SEASON TRAINING

It might appear that the fitness drills you are asked to perform during pre-season over the years are a simply a random mix of lactic acid-creating, vomit-inducing exercises with little structure or specific format.

However, good pre-season sessions are carefully constructed on a week-by-week schedule to condition your body gradually to peak, bang on cue, at the beginning of the season. Badly or incorrectly structured training could leave you open to a range of muscular injuries. You should not be performing too intense training drills too soon.

Start your pre-season training reasonably gently – don't be tempted to include large numbers of repetitive 100 per cent all-out sprints over 30 yards. These sessions are great later on when your fitness levels are high, but putting too much stress on unconditioned leg muscles is like putting a 1000cc motorbike engine on a moped. The frame of the moped is not designed to tolerate that kind of power and, in the same way, your thighs, adductors and hamstrings are not ready for full on maximum intensity sprints – at least, not until a base level of fitness has been established.

Pre-season isn't just about fitness. The skill of the team

manager is to collaborate with his fitness and conditioning staff to ensure players' fitness levels are worked on at the same time as their ball skills. One shouldn't fall behind the other. A player is useless if he has exceptional levels of fitness but dire ball skills and equally useless if he has a golden touch but is blowing out of his rear end after 30 minutes.

Integrating the two disciplines is essential to ensure the team will perform throughout the coming season. Putting too much emphasis on one or the other could be detrimental later on in the season.

As far as the fitness aspect of pre-season is concerned, it can be generally be broken down into a number of categories:

- Aerobic conditioning
- Strength training
- Anaerobic conditioning
- Speed and agility

How long you spend working on each stage very much depends on how long you give yourself to get in shape for the start of the season.

In an ideal world, eight weeks should give you plenty of time to build a level of fitness to leave anyone playing against you for dead. Your body will be able to tolerate the highest intensity of matches and your fitness levels will give you the opportunity to remain focussed and sharp for the full 90 minutes – and beyond.

So why do you need to structure your pre-season fitness

training and what should each stage of the programme actually involve?

AEROBIC CONDITIONING

Before you even start thinking about working on speed and agility, it is essential that you build up a solid aerobic base first.

When the season starts, you're going to need to be able to put in 90 minutes of work, but without the aerobic fitness to be able to keep moving for the full game you're seriously going to start flagging after the first half. Great if you don't mind being substituted at half-time and would actually rather be in the bar before the final whistle blows rather than celebrate a win with your mates... but not so great if you are serious about your performance.

The distance you'll be expected to cover varies greatly from position to position, but you should expect to do somewhere in the region of 5-6 miles over the course of a game. Of course, a portion of that is going to involve light jogging or walking but in a high intensity match, you should factor in to get approximately three seconds of rest for every two minutes of effort. In other words, you will be moving and making your cardiovascular system work to at least 75 per cent of maximum capacity nearly all the time.

Use the first two to three weeks of your pre-season fitness programme to condition your aerobic system. A great litmus test is simply to head out for a 5-6 mile run and see how you get on. Use a heart monitor to get yourself to within the region of 70-75 per cent of your maximum. That's very roughly around 140-150 beats per minute for a 20-year-old, but it's best if you make the calculation based on your true maximum heart rate – as explained in the last chapter.

Struggling to cover the distance at this pace would indicate your aerobic capacity is some way down and you need to do some serious work on conditioning your heart and your slow twitch muscle fibres if you want to give yourself any chance of having a great season.

On the other hand, if you can do the distance at 75 per cent or more, then well done – aerobically, you're in pretty good nick. In fact, the ability to train for any length of time at a heart rate of 80 per cent plus indicates you can already clear low levels of lactic acid from your working muscles and sustain exercise. This means you are starting to run anaerobically.

Don't rely on the 5-6 mile test as your sole method of assessing your aerobic capacity, even if you're very good at it. Don't forget – you're training for football – a stop-start game, not a continuous run at a constant pace. By all means embark on a few five-milers as part of your training but don't waste your weeks of aerobic conditioning on running at the same pace for 45 minutes.

The two best ways of supercharging your aerobic fitness are:

● Fartlek – vary the speed of your 5-6 mile runs
● Perform a series of aerobic conditioning drills
  on the pitch

FARTLEK – THE FOOTBALLER'S FRIEND

Fartlek training is a fantastic way to make your five-milers more specific to football and really set yourself up nicely for the next level up of training.

Fartlek is a Swedish word which means speed play. As the translation suggests, Fartlek training incorporates a series of high intensity bursts within a longer run. In the early part of the pre-season, we're not talking about all-out 100 per cent effort sprints, but rather taking your running pace up from around 60-70 per cent to 80-85 per cent of your maximum speed for 30 seconds or so. Over time, these sessions help the body to build up a tolerance to the accumulation of lactic acid in the working muscles.

Your body or, more specifically, your nervous system can get used to functioning at low running speeds and may react slowly to the commands your brain gives to your legs – which isn't a great characteristic to have as a footballer. By interspersing quicker bursts of pace into your long runs in the form of the Fartlek, you keep that all-important nervous system awake and responsive, strengthen your heart, improve your aerobic capacity and condition yourself nicely for the next part of pre-season.

A word of warning. If you have spent a few weeks of the off-season in Ibiza partying hard and you start pre-season in pretty poor shape, leave the Fartlek sessions alone – at least until you have a couple of gentle four or five-milers under your belt. Start off slowly and gradually build the intensity.

PITCH INVASION – TRAINING ON THE PARK

It's a great idea to start your pre-season training on the paddock itself, if you have easy access to a football field. Let's face it – you're going to be playing on grass, so why not train on it?

Aerobic conditioning on the pitch gets your pre-season fitness regime started. Using a ball during training gives you the opportunity to work on your strength training.

Make sure you have a stopwatch so that you can time working and rest periods to get the most out of your aerobic base-building sessions on the pitch. And take along a heart rate monitor.

There are hundreds of ways to spend the first couple of weeks of pre-season by yourself on the pitch, but the important thing to remember is to keep the intensity relatively low at this stage and not sprint. All you should be looking to do is to keep working at a heart rate max of 70-75 per cent for 20-30 minutes, working up to 45 minutes by the end of the aerobic conditioning period.

An example of a session might be something like this:

● Jog around the pitch for a good 5-10 minutes and stretch the major muscles as explained earlier in the chapter
● Start the session at 75 per cent of your maximum pace up to the halfway line and back again. Wait 30 seconds and repeat. Do this five times
● Your heart rate should average somewhere in the region of 70-80 per cent of your maximum heart rate by the end of the fifth run

- After a short breather and no more than 60 seconds after your fifth interval, dribble a ball at a jogging pace around the pitch twice, speeding up a touch (not sprinting) for ten seconds or so every time you reach a corner flag
- Once you've finished your lap, take a swig of water and repeat the whole session again
- Depending on your heart rate and how you feel, do this circuit three or four times. If your heart rate remains high and you start to feel fatigued, ease the pace right down and make sure you only train at 75-80 per cent of maximum heart rate
- Remember to cool down slowly by jogging around the pitch and stretch well at the end of the session

This type of session can be varied greatly and over the course of a typical three-week period of aerobic conditioning try upping the intensity a little as your fitness levels improve:

- Reduce your recovery time between shuttle runs
- Increase the number of shuttle runs from five to ten
- Increase the speed of your recovery dribble around the park
- Integrate some strength work in between intervals (see next section)

However you choose to increase the intensity of the sessions, never lose sight of your ultimate goal. You are training your heart and the slow twitch muscles in your legs to tolerate long periods of football specific work at a medium intensity. Running intervals too fast at this stage will be too much for your muscles and heart to cope with after a summer of beer abuse on the beaches of the Balearics.

First train your body to work at a 70-80 per cent of maximum effort for 30-40 minutes while integrating dribbling skills and getting your muscles used to playing football again.

STRENGTH TRAINING

I have sandwiched strength training between aerobic and anaerobic conditioning not because you should only perform 2-3 weeks of strength-specific training immediately after your aerobic conditioning, but so you can integrate your strength training at *any* time.

The strength requirements for footballers are nowhere near the same as that of a rugby player. All the same, a certain amount of upper and lower body strength training is vital. Weights sessions in the gym are not generally synonymous with footballers but they can be incredibly useful – if done correctly – in making you dynamically stronger and in adding to your cardiovascular fitness. By increasing your strength by just 10 per cent you will make yourself a 10 per cent better player. Period.

The big question is – how do you go about integrating a strength training workout into your pre-season training? You already have to dedicate most of your time to improving aerobic and anaerobic fitness. And then there is work on speed and agility.

Those players in the Premiership who take their fitness

seriously find the time to hit the gym and work on their strength without difficulty. You, on the other hand, have a full-time job and hardly enough space to fit in your cardio-training, let alone strength training as well. It can be incredibly difficult to integrate a strength building programme.

If you are lucky enough to have the time to fit in a few sessions at the gym to work on your upper body and leg strength, then great, but you can easily build it into your aerobic and anaerobic training sessions – and without using a single dumbbell!

It might sound a little old school, but good old press-ups, lunges, free-standing squats and sit-ups are all fantastic exercises to integrate with your training sessions and you'll be surprised at how much stronger you will feel after just a few sessions. There isn't even any reason why you can't use some of these exercises at the beginning of pre-season, but I'd suggest you do a few aerobic training sessions to get your cardiovascular system into reasonable shape.

If your fitness levels at the start of pre-season are pretty poor and you start performing a series of press-ups and lunges in-between sets of training runs, you'll find that your heart rate will not have time to recover and you'll tire quite quickly. Strength training is important but you don't want to be exhausted just 15 minutes into your first training session. Get your aerobic fitness up first, and then add strength to sessions.

Once you feel your aerobic fitness is at a reasonable level and you are able to train at 70-75 per cent of your maximum heart rate for at least 30 minutes you can start playing around with a few sets of press–ups and squats, etc.

You could start by performing one set of each exercise during your recovery period between running intervals. If we use the previous aerobic training session as an example:

- Jog around the pitch for a good 5-10 minutes and stretch the major muscles as explained earlier in the chapter
- Start the session by running at 75 per cent of your maximum pace to the halfway line and back again. Wait 30 seconds and repeat. Do this five times
- Your heart rate should average somewhere in the region of 70-80 per cent of your maximum by the end of the fifth run
- Take a short breather then instead of taking the ball around the pitch, perform a series of upper body and lower body exercises, such as:
- 20 press-ups performed at a medium tempo
- 20 free-standing squats
- 20 sit-ups
- Take the ball around the pitch, have a swig of water on your return to the starting position and repeat the session over again
- Cool down slowly – jog around the pitch and stretch

As your cardiovascular fitness improves and you start to get stronger, increase the intensity of your sessions. There are a number of ways to go about achieving this. Perform 30 repetitions of each exercise or drop a few different ones into the mix. Over time, your strength gains will be noticeable and you'll be well on the way to being a fitter and stronger player than you were last season.

Take dumbbell sets and a stability ball with you to the training pitch if you really want to make significant strength gains. The versatility of the dumbbells adds a whole new dimension to your strength training programme. You can use them to target a range of muscles, such as the deltoids (shoulders – essential for barging people off the ball) biceps, triceps and back muscles.

The benefits of using a stability ball as part of your strength training are endless. Its unstable properties make it an excellent medium for core strengthening – an area massively overlooked by both amateur and professional players. Although the importance of a strong core is well recognised at Premiership level, the introduction of specific core training has been one aspect of fitness which entered the game surprisingly late. It has only been in the last five years or so that strength and conditioning coaches have made it a mandatory requirement in fitness training regimes.

And just because you are an amateur doesn't mean you should neglect the importance of it yourself. My advice is to make sure that you train the core as part of your aerobic and anaerobic programme. Take a stability ball to the training paddock and integrate some exercises targeting at the core during your recovery between sets.

It's beyond the scope of this book to provide in-depth drills and exercises for the core, but an instructor at your local gym will be able to give you some good advice.

In the meantime, to get you going, try doing press-ups while resting your feet on the stability ball. You may well find this difficult until you have strengthened your core musculature. Then you can make it harder. Do the press-ups with one leg raised up. Keeping yourself stable will really tax the core muscles.

Strength training for football will understandably be near the bottom of your list of priorities as an amateur player with limited time to train and commitments to work, family or study. The pros perform a series of strength drills on the pitch during running sessions but they also have the time to hit the weights in the gym and can draw on expert instruction to properly train muscles. You – sadly – do not have this luxury, so my advice is to utilise your time on the paddock and make your strength training part of your aerobic or anaerobic training.

ANAEROBIC TRAINING

You're ready to turn the intensity up a notch and start training your anaerobic fitness now you've spent a couple of weeks conditioning your aerobic fitness and shaking off the effects of a lazy summer on the beach.

Fitness gains at this stage will help your body build up tolerance to higher levels of lactic acid in the blood and that means you can run at pace for longer. If done correctly, anaerobic training also aids recovery from intense periods of play. The body is better able to clear the acidic waste products which accumulate during those short, sharp bouts of running which are so characteristic of the game and the result will be a dramatic improvement in your performance.

There are a number of different types of anaerobic training but they are all aimed towards the same result. You are looking to train at higher speeds than you can attain through aerobic training and you want to be able to do it with a shorter recovery time. Essentially, you will make your body adapt to the length of time you will be running at pace during a match.

Your anaerobic training drills should be performed with your running pace at around 80-90 per cent of maximum. These sessions are tough and not particularly pleasant but I'm afraid you have to do them if you want to make significant progress. The Premiership boys spend a considerable amount of time working on their anaerobic conditioning and are hooked up to their heart rate monitors every session. Their coaches know exactly how hard they train and what percentage of their maximum heart rate they are working at.

The Polar Team[2] systems are used by most Premiership teams. They track the heart rate of each player which, according to Polar, should be beating at '80-90 per cent of max to improve high speed endurance and anaerobic tolerance'. Players not meeting these training intensities simply receive a bollocking and are told to speed up.

Of course, you are unlikely to be accountable to anyone if you are not putting the effort into these anaerobic sessions. Your coach may very well put you through some anaerobic training drills at your club, but he's unlikely to keep exact tabs on your level of effort and exercising heart rate. You won't have the luxury of getting a kick up the arse to make you train harder.

Aerobic sessions are for the large part tolerable and, although fatiguing in the final stages, not painful. Anaerobic training sessions hurt – a lot. The longer the sessions last, the harder they get, the more nauseous you feel and the more willpower it takes to complete the session at the necessary intensity.

Whether you train on your own, with a mate or with your club, you have to take responsibility for the amount of effort you put into your anaerobic training session and fight the overwhelming desire to drop the intensity or make up excuses to stop early. The work you put into these sessions will ultimately define you as a player for the season as it means the difference between flagging at important times of key matches and being able to keep up with the pace of the game.

Your aerobic training may very well give you the physical ability to be able to last a full 90 minutes of football, but your anaerobic training will allow you to do play at pace and without fatigue – get it right and you'll be laughing.

You are going to have to dedicate a good three weeks of hard training to really make a significant improvement in your anaerobic fitness. Start off gently – do not embark on your first training session over-enthusiastically.

The key point to remember during these sessions is to keep focused on what your physiological goal is – i.e., to train the body to adapt to high-intensity running and recover quickly between periods of high intensity work. Therefore, your anaerobic training should wholeheartedly encourage bucket-loads of lactic acid to pour into your muscles so that your body can adapt and learn to get rid of it.

There are hundreds of different training drills you can do to improve your anaerobic capacity but as time to train is likely to be limited, I'd suggest you integrate some strength training in the latter stages of your anaerobic programme.

At this stage of the pre-season in an ideal world you should be training on the pitch. There might be occasions where this is not possible and you'll have to fit a training session at the gym or out running on the road. And while this type of training isn't as specific as that performed on the training pitch, it doesn't mean it's not useful.

FARTLEKING FOR REAL MEN

Okay, so you might have played around with some Fartlek sessions for your aerobic preparations and discovered that, if done properly, this varying paced training is pretty uncomfortable.

Well, that was girl's stuff.

Performing a Fartlek training session over a five-mile run with the specific goal of conditioning your anaerobic fitness is tough and, if you're doing it on your own, requires mental strength to keep you going through the session without dropping the intensity or having to extend your recovery time.

If you've performed Fartlek runs for the aerobic conditioning stage of pre-season or indeed during quick sections of training on the pitch then you will already have been entering an anaerobic state of training for short periods of time. Not high end anaerobic training, but anaerobic training, nonetheless.

Now your quick intervals should be run for no longer than 60 seconds with the aim of working towards shorter bursts of 20 or 30 seconds – but all performed at a far quicker pace than those you did earlier in pre-season.

As for recovery periods between intervals, be strict with yourself and do not allow more time because you are still tired.

This is the whole point of anaerobic training!

An example of a Fartlek training run over five miles:

- Head out for a five-mile run, jogging nice and easily for the first five minutes
- Stop and have a stretch (dynamically, to wake up the nervous system) and get ready for some serious discomfort
- Stopwatch ready, head out again at a jogging pace and after a few minutes, when you feel mentally ready, start your Fartlek intervals
- Start your stopwatch and increase your pace to 80 per cent of maximum speed for 60 seconds
- Recover by either walking or slow jogging for 60 seconds
- Repeat the same interval at the same pace and same recovery time
- Aim to do this five or six times initially, building up to eight times as your fitness levels improve

You don't need me to tell you that these sessions are really tough but they are incredible for turning you into a running machine once the season begins. The key thing to remember is that you are in your anaerobic training now, so dropping your pace to a measly 70 per cent of maximum speed for your 'quick' interval is not good enough and not effective at maximising anaerobic fitness.

As your fitness improves over the three or so weeks of anaerobic training of performing these intervals, increase the intensity by reducing the recovery time by ten seconds. This will further encourage your body to adapt to accumulating volumes of lactic acid in the muscles and will make you more resistant to fatigue after high-intensity training.

In the final stages of this section of pre-season, you can further develop your Fartlek sessions in order to better condition your fast twitch muscle fibres.

Why not try running for 30 seconds at 90 per cent of your maximum pace and following that with 30 seconds of recovery? Performing this quicker Fartlek session up to 15 times requires great determination and willpower to keep pushing yourself to complete the session, but the fitness gains to be made are immense.

ANAEROBIC TRAINING ON THE PITCH

If you can do the bulk of your anaerobic training on the pitch your leg muscles will better become used to running on grass – as opposed to concrete – and you will be able to integrate some ball skills between training sets.

I could spend the next hundred pages giving you sample

training drills but, by now, from what you have learned about anaerobic training and a little bit about heart rate training, you should be able to devise your own routines. As long as you remember that your training heart rate should be over 80 per cent at running speed and your pace is somewhere around 85-90 per cent of your maximum, you can devise whatever training routine you wish.

A tip though.

You're not that far away from the beginning of the season and so you've got to start thinking about making your training as match-specific as possible. Incorporate backwards running, practicing shadowing as part of your drill. This will recruit muscles different to those used in running forwards, so it's essential that you train them during pre-season so that they are conditioned for match situations. Equally important to include in the run are zigzag runs, lateral runs and, to prepare for doing headers, a few jumps.

An example of a typical anaerobic session could go something like this:

- Jog around the pitch for a good 5-10 minutes and stretch the major muscles as explained earlier in the chapter
- Now jog around the pitch a couple of times at a faster pace, dribbling a ball, getting progressively quicker
- As soon as you return to your starting point, you should be well warmed up and your heart rate should be up. Take a breather of no more than 30 seconds and have a drink

- Start the session with a fast run at 85 per cent of your maximum pace to the halfway line and back again. Wait 30 seconds and repeat. Do this six times
- Vary the exercise. Change running direction every now and again or run backwards for ten yards once in a while
- Your heart rate should be somewhere in the region of 90 per cent of your maximum heart rate by the end of the sixth run
- After a short breather and no more than 60 seconds after your sixth interval, dribble a ball at a jogging pace around the pitch twice
- Take a swig of water and repeat the whole session again
- Remember to cool down slowly by jogging around the pitch and stretch well at the end of the session

Depending on your heart rate and how you feel, do this circuit three times with variations. Integrate some strength training drills during your intervals in the shape of jump squats, press-ups or sit-ups at the end of each interval. In the early stages of your anaerobic training this may be too intense but when you're ready you really should introduce some form of upper body training.

As you progress through the anaerobic training part of pre-season, vary the training intensity by reducing your recovery time and adding more intervals to each session. If you fail to do this, you will not improve and you won't be making the most of your training.

SPEED AND AGILITY

The final few weeks of pre-season training should see you concentrating on developing your speed and agility. You may well have had a good turn of pace at the end of last season, but it's amazing what a summer off can do to your fast twitch muscles if they haven't been used. The last three or so weeks of pre-season should be used to wake up your fast twitch muscle fibres and get them to contract at lightning-quick pace as soon as they receive the 'sprint' message from your brain.

Speed and agility training will specifically target those explosive muscle fibres which are responsible for you covering 50 yards as quickly as possible. Your nervous system will become more responsive and this will help to improve your reaction time.

Speed and agility is the favoured form of training for most players as it gives you a licence to really put your foot down and run at pace and the sensation gives you a real buzz. But as essential a part of pre-season at it is, you should first have followed the stages of conditioning to ensure your heart, lungs and muscles are already in good enough shape to be able to tolerate the stresses that sprinting places on the body. When running flat out, especially from a standing start, your tendons and muscle fibres are under immense tension and it is so easy to injure yourself.

Interestingly, to highlight this point, research carried out by the FA found that the month with the greatest number of injuries was July – out of season, during training. The reasons for this are, of course, varied, but I'd strongly suggest that it can at least in part be explained by players taking time off training for the summer and returning with the expectation that their bodies can tolerate the same degree of exertion as they did at the end of the season.

Always make sure you have a good fitness base before you return to the same intensity of exercise and, even then, be careful and work up gradually.

So what is the best way to train for speed? Run a few 100-metre intervals?

Definitely not, argues my fitness contact within the Premiership: 'What's the point in training the body to run repeated intervals of 100 metres at maximum pace,' he says, 'when you're not going to be running that far and that quick during a game?'

No matter if you play in the Premiership or the Sunday league, there is no point in wasting valuable training time on training sessions which won't help to improve your football fitness.

During the vast majority of full pace sprints in a typical competitive game you will cover no more than 40 yards or so before taking a break. Of course, you may very well have to cover another rapid 40 yards about 20 seconds later, but repeatedly training over 100 metres is largely unnecessary and counterproductive. When you consider that the average all-out sprint in a game lasts no longer than two seconds you soon realise how unimportant it is to sprint over much longer distances.

The key to developing your speed is to perform a series of short sharp sprints (no longer than ten seconds) lots of times

– resting between sets. You may want to sprint from the goal line to the edge of the penalty area, rest for ten seconds and repeat four or five times – then take a long break. You'll find that if you try to perform too many sprints your creatine phosphate levels will not have enough time to recover and you'll simply be unable to run at the all-important, 100 per cent flat-out rate. You may very well be making anaerobic fitness gains by performing numerous sprints (albeit with the latter intervals run closer to 90 per cent of max pace) but you won't be training for speed, which is what this part of pre-season is all about.

As your speed fitness improves and your leg muscles become stronger, faster and more efficient at recovering from your high intensity sprints, then you can start to reduce your recovery time and perhaps even add a few extra intervals – just make sure you run each interval at 100 per cent of your maximum pace.

Premiership players at this stage of the season will often follow a highly specific weight training programme in conjunction with sprint training to maximise and strengthen the recruitment of the fast twitch muscle fibres of the legs.

Carefully-monitored weight training sessions in which the legs are trained under resistance and every movement is performed at speed are highly effective at improving the function of fast twitch muscle fibres. If they're done incorrectly, however, they can easily lead to injury or even speed reduction.

I strongly suggest you give it a miss – unless you are already familiar with this form of training – and instead focus on performing sprint intervals instead. The Premiership boys will not only have done this form of training for years but, more often than not, will do it under the strict supervision of their fitness and conditioning team.

There are hundreds of variations you can do, as with anaerobic training drills. Follow the basic guidelines and perform your sprints for no longer than ten seconds (preferably somewhere in the 5-8 second bracket) and avoid doing too many intervals before a long break. You'll condition your sprinting muscles perfectly ready for the start of the season.

The final aspect of sprint training which you must not forget to integrate into your sessions is sprinting in different directions. There are going to be plenty of occasions in a match where you'll be expected to sprint one way for a few seconds before suddenly changing your running angle. Your brain and muscles need to be conditioned to react and tolerate this sudden movement, so make sure that a number of your training runs involve a change in direction every now and again – all at pace!

An example of a sprint session:

● Jog around the pitch for a good ten minutes (even 15 minutes on a cold day to ensure your muscles are really nice and warm) and perform a good stretch on all the major muscles
● Jog faster around the pitch a couple of times, dribbling a ball and getting progressively quicker

● As soon as you return to your starting point, you should be well warmed up and your heart rate should be at a good rate

● Start the session with a gentle jog from the goal line to the edge of the penalty area, getting progressively quicker. As soon as you reach the line, sprint at 100 per cent of your maximum pace up to the halfway line, then jog slowly to the edge of the opposite penalty area, finishing off with a sprint to the far goal line

● Wait 30 seconds and repeat. Do this five times, take a few minutes off and do it all over again

● Vary this routine. Change running direction by 45 degrees every now and again

● Your heart rate should be somewhere in the region of 95 per cent of your maximum heart rate by the end of the final run

● Remember to cool down slowly by jogging around the pitch and stretch well at the end of the session

Feel free to play around with this sort of session as much as you like, but at this stage of the season it's best if you perform all of your training on the pitch rather than on the roads.

Always remember to vary the sessions by performing different distance sprints and gradually reduce your recovery time as your fitness improves.

By the end of your third week of this type of training, your leg muscles, heart and mental attitude should be in the perfect place to start the season. Provided you have followed all of the aerobic, anaerobic and sprint training procedures outlined in this chapter you have my word that you will be the fittest you have ever been and physically so well-conditioned that you'll be amazed at what your body can do.

The Premiership contingent may very well be ahead of you in terms of their genetic ability, the amount of time they have spent training at the intensities outlined in this chapter and their access to professional fitness advice, but ultimately they use the very same training techniques as described above.

If you make it your mission that this season you are going to be the fittest you have ever been and dedicate a lot of time and effort to make your pre-season training sessions the most productive ever, you will do amazing things on the pitch for the rest of the season. Your heart, your muscles and your lungs will be able to tolerate the fitness demands of any game, leaving you more able to concentrate on your ball skills, your ability to make and create space for your team-mates and in the process you will sculpt a physique to be proud of.

But it's not just the training which you need to be focusing on – you also need to think about what goes in your mouth. Training and nutrition go together like Ant and Dec, so if you are serious about performing well this season, you need to eat like the pros.

CHAPTER FOUR
FEEDING THE MACHINE
PERFORMANCE-ENHANCING NUTRITION

'Seriously, I was the only player at Ajax who used to have fried eggs for breakfast every day. It's one of my superstitions. If I don't have a fried breakfast in the morning, I won't play or train well.'

Not the words you'd expect to hear in a post-match interview from a top-class footballer these days, but this proclamation from Marc Overmars, the legendary Dutch winger known for his speed and guile, may surprise you.

Although we can safely say that his take on optimum sports nutrition at the highest level is unlikely to be advocated by any of today's Premiership nutritional experts, his penchant for fried eggs certainly didn't appear to affect his ability to play the game at a high standard.

When you look at this example, that someone who represented his country 86 times, scoring 17 goals and earning the nick name 'Road Runner', you'd be forgiven for taking the view that fried eggs on the morning of a game is the perfect performance-enhancing meal and should be adopted by all players.

But while a fry-up may have suited Overmars' superstition, I'm willing to bet that his diet for the rest of the time did not consist of products high in fat and sugar and even if it did, imagine the player he could have been if he'd eaten properly! Interestingly, Ajax were pretty hot on the importance of nutrition in performance, so I would speculate that Overmars' team-mates would not have followed his lead.

Argentinean legend Ossie Ardiles, seen by some to be one of the game's finest-ever players, tells of the time he arrived at Tottenham Hotspur in 1978 and how things have moved on: 'When I arrived, the boys would eat all sorts – I ate steak and chips before a game – and they would all go out for a drink afterwards. I wanted to fit in, so I joined them. Now it is completely different.'

These revelations by Overmars and Ardiles clearly demonstrate just how much attitudes towards the importance of nutrition for players have changed in the past few decades.

In years gone by, the best footballers in the country were pretty much given free rein about what to eat and any advice were given would be laughed off the pitch now by anyone who has a basic understanding of modern nutrition, to say nothing of the professional viewpoint.

For example, it wasn't that long ago that a good chunk of meat such as a steak or pork chop was thought to be just the ticket for feeding the machine in the hours leading up to a big game.

To many people, the logic behind this might sound reasonable:

Steak and chops are high in protein; players use their muscles (made of protein) a lot during an intense game, so the best way to fuel those muscles is by eating lots of protein thereby giving them energy.

This thinking in sports nutrition was followed by players and coaches for years and it is only fairly recently that nutritional science has made dramatic discoveries about what actually fuels the human body during intense sports such as football.

This research, along with the desire of every club to be at the cutting edge of performance enhancement, has lead to a huge overhaul in attitude towards what players eat. Elite players now work and eat under the strict guidance of a team of dieticians and nutritionists who will all stress the importance of eating the right foods at the right time and in the right quantities to get the most out of the player's body and to perform at their maximum potential.

Dieticians and nutritionists go into great detail with each player about the kind of food they should eat. The pros of old would doubtless have found it all pretty laughable as they tucked into their pre-match meal of steak-and-ale pie – but there is no escaping the difference that proper nutrition can make to athletic performance.

FUELLING THE MORTAL MACHINE

So, what can you do to have any hope of following the nutritional tips and secrets of the best that the Premiership has to offer?

The information covered in this chapter will give you an insight into how the pros eat for performance and how you can replicate it at home. Much of what we will be covering is not rocket science but drilling yourself on what and how much of certain types of foods to eat is essential if you truly want to get the best out of your body.

This chapter will give you all the nutritional information you have ever wanted to know about what the Lampards and Beckhams of this world eat in the run-up to and aftermath of a game. Follow the tips and eat the same essential nutrients to fuel your body to play the best game of your life and you'll still have the energy to score in extra time.

For you – the part-time-yet-football-obsessed player – I will give an outline of performance food and supplements which are specific to the needs of the game of football. Many other books on the shelves will give detailed advice on the generic topic of sports nutrition but little accurate nutritional recommendations for the highly specific nature of a 90-minute, explosive and stop-start sport. What you read in the following pages is written for footballers and footballers alone and is all based on what years of research has discovered on what helps players get the very best out of their bodies.

Everything you read is based on what Premiership footballers eat and use to supplement their diets in order to be the best in the country – you'd be crazy to follow any other advice so enjoy learning how to 'fuel the machine'.

THE BASICS OF EATING FOR ENERGY: CARBOHYDRATES ARE KING!

As already discussed, the role of nutrition in top-flight football has changed dramatically since the 1970s.

In the later part of that decade, theory and unsubstantiated ideas from various nutritional studies hardened into fact. It became clear there was a distinct relationship between eating properly and improving player performance. This breakthrough eventually made some of the highest profile and most resilient coaches – who were reluctant to embrace change – adopt a more favourable view of how eating particular foods could mean the difference between winning and losing.

A classic example of how coaching attitudes have altered towards health and nutrition since the '70s can be found in an incident involving legendary manager Brain Clough. At the time, Cloughy was a novice manager of second division Derby County and was about to play host to first division team Leeds United (how times have changed) in the FA Cup. Cloughy, desperate to make a good impression, prepared a little welcome pack for the Leeds players which included neatly folded towels, the obligatory orange and... a glass ashtray!

As generous as this sentiment may have been at the time, nearly 40 years later a repeat of this gesture would have poor Cloughy needing to have an ashtray surgically removed from where the sun don't shine after a likely fracas with the Leeds United manager not taking kindly to his 'hospitable' gesture.

Managers of today are so much stricter on what they allow their players to put in their mouth that the mere mention of a post-match fag would probably invite a hefty fine or one almighty bollocking.

Back in the late '70s and early '80s, at a time when the league was slowly growing in financial stature and winning led to more valuable rewards than bragging rights, the men in charge of the teams changed their stance and took a far more serious view of the role of nutrition in the game.

So what made them change their minds and how much of an impact did it have on a player's ability to perform better?

To try and isolate one specific piece of nutritional science research which changed the eating habits of every Premiership player would be sensationalist and not completely true.

A combination of factors over a period of time enforced a change in attitudes in the Premiership. They included science and, perhaps more intriguingly, the influx of foreign players from Europe which followed a dramatic change in European legislation.

In the mid-'90s, the 'Bosman ruling' banned restrictions on foreign European Union (EU) members within the national leagues and allowed professional football players in the EU to move freely to another club at the end of their term of contract with their present team. This led to a dramatic increase in the number of footballers from abroad playing in England and they brought with them cutting-edge theories on eating for performance.

So, you may very well give the pasta-munchers of Italy some friendly abuse when they are playing against England in the World Cup but they are partly responsible for imparting their superior knowledge about eating correctly for better performance.

FOOTBALLERS DON'T DO THE ATKINS

The most valuable piece of advice that the Italians brought with them was the discovery of the effect that carbohydrates had on the working muscles. It changed the eating habits of footballers in the UK.

Even if you know only very little about the best way to feed yourself in order to excel over a 90-minute game of football, you are bound to have heard plenty about carbohydrates.

Did you know that 55-65 per cent of the energy our body uses to play football comes from carbohydrate?

So much attention has been given to carbohydrate-rich foods both in sports nutrition and general health nutrition over the years that many people are left confused as to whether they are beneficial or detrimental to our health. Dr Atkins – the meat-and-fat loving scientist – created a sea of controversy back in the '70s and then again in the early 2000s with his world-famous diet. He advised those who followed his plan to cut out all forms of carbohydrates if they wished to lose weight.

This approach to nutrition has been a controversial way of losing weight but interestingly some of Dr Atkins' theories were followed by some footballers in the past.

The Atkins diet promotes taking a high percentage of your

daily food allowance from fat and protein – and very little from carbohydrate. This dietary approach is not a million miles away from the old-school belief that the best way to energise yourself before a game is to eat pork chops – high in protein – in order to feed the working muscles.

Research in nutrition for human performance has demonstrated that a diet predominately consisting of protein in preparation for an intense bout of exercise lasting 90 minutes is far from ideal and in many cases can actually be detrimental to performance.

A working knowledge of basic sports nutrition will help you understand why this is and why football's elite now eats very differently. To perform at your peak you should have an overview into the way the body is fuelled for movement and how you can give yourself the best chance to last the full 90 minutes and beyond.

Essentially, carbohydrate in the body (pasta, rice, potatoes, etc) is stored as *glycogen* and then converted to *glucose*.

THE BRAIN, GLUCOSE AND THE FOOTBALLER

The very existence of brains in many top-class footballers has been a subject of debate for many years, particularly in the major tabloids, but if nothing else the brain is essential in orchestrating many essential nutritional functions.

Whatever your opinion on the content of a Premiership footballer's brain, it is an essential nutritional organ in the body and requires a steady supply of fuel to keep it alive and functioning optimally. If the supply of glucose is interrupted

– due to illness or its lack in the bloodstream – the brain will simply not be able to function properly and a player may experience a number of symptoms. These can seriously affect his judgement and ability to play anywhere near his best. Such symptoms include:

● Confusion
● Dizziness
● Lethargy
● Inability to concentrate
● Heavy legs

These symptoms clearly have a massive influence on a player's ability to help the team win a tight game. The effect of a low supply of glucose to the brain can quite easily mean the difference between winning and losing.

MUSCLES, GLUCOSE AND THE FOOTBALLER

Feeding the brain the correct amount of glucose is next to useless unless the working muscles can be provided with glucose on tap to contract explosively.

When the brain sends a message to leg it, jump or take a dive, the muscles instantaneously contract and, provided you have enough glucose in the bloodstream, the muscles will do exactly what you tell them to do. How fast they contract depends on how much specific training you have been doing.

The process by which glucose fires muscles into action is beyond the scope of this book. I'll leave pyruvate, the

Krebs cycle and mitochondria to the science bods to explain to you elsewhere. For now, take it from me that if you want to have any chance of improving your game through nutrition, you should feed your muscles enough glucose through complex carbs such as spuds, pasta, rice, etc, to react explosively on demand.

So, how do the nutritionists at the top clubs make sure that players have a steady supply of glucose in the bloodstream to feed the brain and muscles the nutrients they need to function properly?

It's all about utilising the body's ability to store large amounts of carbohydrate which can then be broken down and converted into glucose to be used as and when required.

Without this storage capacity players would not be able to last ten minutes – let alone the full 90. It is essential that you ensure that your internal stores of carbohydrate are sufficient to last you the game.

STORING CARBOHYDRATES IN THE BODY

The ability to store carbohydrates in the body is not one that we directly control, though there are a number of ways in which we can influence it – at least that is the case for most people. Sadly, as Tottenham hero Gary Mabbutt discovered at the age of just 17, the ability to store carbohydrates in muscles and liver should not be taken for granted. He had been experiencing odd symptoms such as excessive thirst and general lethargy and finally realised during a competitive game something was not right. Yet he struggled on to complete the match, feeling sluggish and exhausted, and decided it was time he got checked out. After just five minutes with the doctor, Mabbutt was diagnosed with Type 1 diabetes. He was told he was unable to produce insulin, the hormone ultimately responsible for storing carbohydrates in the muscles.

The body's ability to store and provide essential carbohydrates to the working brain and muscles during exercise has been the subject of many studies. They concluded that, once eaten, complex carbohydrates such as rice, pasta and potatoes are broken down with the help of digestive enzymes so the body can transport them in the blood. The body's internal regulation system then automatically directs sugar to the areas where it is needed.

The body stores carbohydrate in your muscles and your liver in the form of a substance known as glycogen so that you don't need to keep eating carbohydrates every hour of the day to meet the body's demand. It was a deeper understanding about the ability to store glycogen that led coaches and conditioning staff to seriously review the way they used food to make players play faster for longer.

Whether you are Frank Lampard, John Terry, Theo Walcott or just someone who hacks around on a Wednesday evening with your mates, you are reliant on your body's internal glycogen store to keep your legs moving.

Without a sufficient supply, both your physical performance and mental state of mind will be severely compromised and will slowly grind to a halt.

THE IMPORTANCE OF GLYCOGEN

The human body can store somewhere in the region of 500 grams (1.1 pounds) of carbohydrate in the form of glycogen, 100 grams of which is stored in the liver and 400 grams in the muscles. This is enough to keep you running for about two hours, although the figure will vary enormously depending on your musculature, how fast you run and your own individuality.

Once those stores start to run low, the body relies more heavily on alternative stores of energy – such as fat and protein – to keep movement sustained. The process of converting fat and protein into quick energy is complex and the body is unable to do it fast enough to meet the explosive energy demands of the game, which ultimately leads to deterioration in performance.

If carbohydrate stores remain low there will be an insufficient supply of sugar available to keep the brain working properly. This gives rise to symptoms of dizziness and confusion. If you continue exercising with these symptoms your health can deteriorate very quickly. You can collapse and fall ill. This drop in blood sugar is known as hypoglycaemia and is explained in more detail later.

It would be incredibly unlikely for a Premiership player to suffer from low glycogen levels. If low carb stores were to lead to poor performance then the player – or the dietician – would swiftly feel the full force of the manager's foot hitting their arse. It is the expert's responsibility to ensure players take on enough carbohydrate.

A certain amount of glycogen is of great importance in any

sport played at high intensity, but as far as football is concerned it is not essential to load muscles and liver to their maximum capacity. What might well be of use to a marathon runner – whose stores will be depleted around mile 18 – is a hindrance for a footballer. The extra weight that great stocks of glycogen add to the body is surplus to requirements and could impede performance.

All this information is all well and good but you still have to know exactly how much carbohydrate you should eat to maximise your performance.

Can you have too much?

How do you know if you are eating enough?

Premiership players have the luxury of access to nutritional experts who analyse their exact carbohydrate requirements based on such factors as biochemical individuality and precise exercise demands. But all is not lost for the rest of us.

It is far harder to get the levels exactly right, but by using basic principles described later on, you too can regulate your carbohydrate intake to maximise your endurance capacity on the park.

TIMING CARBOHYDRATE INTAKE

Sadly, to put a spanner in the works, ensuring that you have sufficient carbohydrate to train and play a full-on, high-intensity match without running out of gas is not quite as simple as you may think. Unlike refuelling a car where you just fill up and go, the timing of your carbohydrate intake is vital.

Taking on carbohydrates too close to the kick off of a game

may lead to stomach cramps and stitches, but leave too much time and the drop in blood sugar levels might leave you lethargic and sluggish.

Timing is essential due to the role of enzymes in the body responsible for carbohydrate management.

The body secretes large amounts of an enzyme called glycogenase immediately after exercise. It makes the muscles and liver highly receptive to the absorption and storage of carbohydrate. The level of glycogenase in the blood is raised for about two hours – the optimum window for replacement of lost carbohydrate stores. Numerous studies have been performed on this subject and the evidence is overwhelmingly in favour of consuming a rich carbohydrate meal or drink soon after training or a match. If insufficient carbohydrate is eaten or it is taken in at the wrong time, performance can be severely compromised in subsequent training sessions or even matches. You might not even realise why you feel so tired.

Players drink copious amounts of sports drinks after a game not just to replace lost fluids but also to replace lost sugars and to start the process of carbohydrate restocking. When the players get out of the changing rooms they will eat a meal rich in carbohydrates to replenish burned off energy and restock it ready for next time. And did you know Premiership clubs see this post-match carbohydrate replenishment as being so important that they prepare just the right amount of carb rich foods for player to take immediately after the game?

The details vary from club to club, but most encourage players to eat around 300 grams of carbohydrates straight after the game. To make this practical, meals are prepared in 50-gram portions in the form of wraps, pasta, carbohydrate drinks, etc.

There is no reason why you too can't follow the same procedure...

PRE-MATCH MEAL: TO CARB OR NOT TO CARB?

At the beginning of the chapter I highlighted the fact that there was a time when the likes of Argentinean legend Ossie Ardiles used to eat steak and chips before a match.

Eating the right thing on the day of a match these days is essential to ensure that you perform well in the park. You may very well have religiously followed an individualised and highly detailed nutritional programme in the week leading up to the game, but eat the wrong thing at the wrong time in the run up and your guts could be in for some serious trouble.

If pre-match nerves alone are enough to churn the stomach before a game – add a meal which is either difficult to digest or which goes straight through you and you'll end up doubled over with a stitch or even worse – the inexorable desire to run off the pitch and find the nearest toilet.

Not surprisingly, when it comes to pre-match meals, it is often a case of different strokes for different folks. One meal may not necessarily suit all players. If you are intolerant to wheat, for example, a plate of pasta three hours before a match will not really be the smartest option to choose.

The guidelines for selecting the most appropriate food apply as much to you as they do to Premiership players. Just because they are better players than you doesn't mean that they need a posher or super-scientific meal to make them play well.

Scientifically, there are a few rules which you should bear in mind when deciding what to eat before a match:

RULE ONE: DON'T LEAVE IT TOO LATE

Timing your pre-match meal correctly is essential for performance.

If you leave it too late and start exercising too soon after eating, blood is diverted away from the digestive system to feed the working muscles instead. This leaves undigested food in your stomach which can lead to crippling stitches and have a massive impact on your performance.

If you eat too soon and start with a hint of the munchies, there is a chance that your blood sugar levels could drop, leaving you with reduced energy to train or play.

The exact timing of pre-match meal varies from person to person, but it is generally recognised that you should eat around two to three hours before the match. The closer you are until kick off, the smaller the meal should be

RULE TWO: EAT SOMETHING FAMILIAR

Experimenting with new delicacies before a match is not recommended. Always stick to a meal you know your stomach is able to tolerate. Leave the vindaloo or sushi for post-match and instead opt for something which you have eaten since you were a kid. You will know your stomach will not react badly.

RULE THREE: CARB UP?

Although some argue against eating large amount of carbohydrate before a game, it is generally advised that in order to ensure your glycogen levels are sufficient to see you through a game, a meal of 50-60 per cent carbohydrate is recommended. This is especially so if previous meals have not been of high quality. For example, you might be running late, miss a decent breakfast and then have a low carb lunch. You won't have had much carbohydrate for a good 18 hours. This is more than enough time for your body to use its internal stores to fuel normal physiological functions and, once the whistle blows at 2pm, you could quite easily see yourself in all kinds of trouble by half-time.

Always use your own judgement when it comes to deciding how much carbohydrate to eat before a game – fuelling pre-match is an individual thing, so think before you eat. It's a subject much debated by food science boffins – when one theory is presented, it often seems to be almost immediately dismissed by other researchers.

For example, some say that the increase of insulin brought on by a carbohydrate-rich meal before a game could be detrimental to performance. It suppresses the utilisation of fat, thereby accelerating the oxidation (use) of carbohydrate for exercise. This causes blood sugar levels to drop. Yet there are those in the scientific community who say that performance is not affected as long as there is enough carbohydrate in the body in the first place.

All in all, it is a very complex subject. One which the

Premiership players don't have to think about but, unfortunately, you do.

If nothing else, use your common sense and resist the temptation to always eat what a friend eats or you could end up spending the first half seeing nothing but the door of the cubicle.

CARBOHYDRATE REQUIREMENTS

Determining exactly how much carbohydrate you should eat daily to meet your exercise demands is really tricky if you don't have your own personal dietician or nutritionist. Our individual requirements for exercise vary so much and even two players who are the same weight and fitness may well find different levels of carbohydrate suit their bodies.

Although it might sound over-the-top to those of you whose pre-match (and possibly post-match) meal of choice is a Cornish pasty and a pint of Fosters, the elite players of this country have all been physiologically analysed in detail. As the modern game at the professional level has got more serious, so has attention to detail about every aspects of nutrition – and that is especially true of carbohydrate intake.

The elite players have their individual resting metabolic rates assessed along with their heart rate response in training and their VO2 max. The professionals' nutritionists know exactly how much energy each player expends at rest as well as during training and therefore how much carbohydrate they need to eat to replenish lost stores. So if you want to play like Stevie G then start by thinking twice about tucking into pie-and-chips after pre-season training –

or at least first find out how many carb calories you are shovelling down in the process.

How do you know how much carbohydrate you should eat without access to professional help? How can you avoid making the schoolboy error of thinking that just because you are training like a banshee you can get away with eating like a horse? It's not a justification to say that you 'are in training for the season'.

Firstly, get these statistics about energy expenditure into your mind – and remember them next time you prepare a carb-rich meal.

- It is thought that most top players run somewhere in the region of seven miles in a match, with many believing that David Beckham covered nearer ten miles in his one-man performance against Greece in 2001
- Seven miles of running over a 90-minute game of football, running at a fast average pace of 7.5 miles an hour (12.1 kilometres an hour) will, give or take, help you expend somewhere in the region of 14 calories a minute
- Approximately 60-70 per cent of this expended energy will come from carbohydrate stores
- Roughly speaking, then, you will burn over 1200 calories during a match – with 700-800-plus of those calories coming from your glycogen stores

There's your answer. In order to fuel your body to tear around the pitch for 90 minutes like a bat out of hell, assuming a total average pace of 7.5 miles an hour, then all you need to do is to wolf down not far off a kilogram of pasta or rice prior to the match and you'll have more energy than a sex-starved nymphomaniac? Right?

Well... not exactly.

Sports nutrition and, certainly, individual carbohydrate metabolism is complex. More complex than any woman – and far more unpredictable (if that's possible).

The stats above, although correct in principle and applicable to a 70 kilogram male, cannot be applied to everyone. If they could, then sports nutritionists would be out of a job and we'd all be able to eat like Premiership stars. By all means use the above generic information to act as a guide but you'd be foolish to follow it to the letter.

For example, although the carbohydrate required for playing a game at an average pace of 7.5 miles an hour (which is damn quick incidentally) is the equivalent of nearly one kilogram of rice, you've got to consider that your body already stores a lot of glycogen without loading up with extras. The remnants of your breakfast, fruit snacks, yesterday's lunch, etc will all be stored away in your muscles and liver, drip-feeding your bloodstream with glucose to feed your brain and working muscles – even when they're idle.

This is where the luxury of having your own nutritionist really comes into its own. With a nutritionist to tell you exactly how much energy you expend every day and how much food you eat, it is far easier to tweak your dietary programme once in a while to ensure you have the exact number of useable calories to train and play.

CARBING UP THE PREMIERSHIP WAY

So how do the pros do it?

Well, take a random Premiership superstar such as Frank Lampard for example. When he first joined Chelsea, his club at the time of writing, he would have been fully physiologically assessed to find out his resting metabolic rate (RMR). This can be done in a number of ways and, as science develops, so do testing protocols. However, one method would involve him taking a day off training before the test and then fasting over that night. In a temperature-controlled environment a series of physiological tests would be performed on him to determine his RMR. Although the intricate details of this test can be quite complex, it's essentially performed to gather information about how much heat Frank's body emits at rest.

The sports science geeks can then work out how many calories he burns while doing nothing – or, put simply, how much energy his muscles, brain and internal organs need in order to function properly. For most people like you and me, this figure is somewhere between 2500 and 2700 calories daily but for top-level athletes it can be much higher.

RMR anyway varies greatly depending on sex (women have lower RMRs), individual genetics and – key to athletes such as Mr Lampard – muscle mass. Due to the fact that muscle is a metabolically-active tissue requiring a large number of calories to survive even at rest, it follows that the more muscle mass you have, the more calories you need to take on board.

Top class players like Frank Lampard will have a higher

RMR than your average amateur player and need somewhere in excess of 3000-3500 calories just to live and maintain their physique – and so that figure goes up when you factor in training time.

How does RMR help to work out how many carbs the elite should eat?

Well, you'll have realised it gives the nutrition team a good idea of how many calories their players need before they've even taken one step on the training field. From this, and after collaboration with exercise scientists who work out how much energy players expend running at certain intensities, the nutritionists can paint a very accurate picture indeed of how many carb calories each player needs individually to have enough energy to train, play a match and maintain a good body weight.

It is a very delicate balance which is predominantly overseen by the team to ensure players have enough energy to train while at the same time not eating an excessive amount of carbohydrate. This avoids gathering the sort of surplus which would be converted into body fat and lead to shouts of 'Who ate all the pies?' from the stands.

CARBING UP THE SUNDAY LEAGUE WAY

You are far less equipped than your Premiership colleagues to work out how much carbohydrate you need to eat to fuel your body to play the beautiful game.

Luckily for you, you're reading this book, because the following information could help to revolutionise your game and put you one step ahead of your opposite number.

STEP ONE: BOOK AN APPOINTMENT WITH A
FITNESS/PERSONAL TRAINER

But not just any trainer. Before you make an appointment, make sure that he or she has access to a Bodystat machine – the next best thing to a lab designed to measure your RMR.

Bodystat uses technology called bioelectrical impedance to analyse your body composition by, effectively, sending an electrical pulse from an electrode attached to your fingers to another electrode attached to your toe. Totally painless, this electrical pulse collects data about your body composition to give the trainer priceless information which you can take home to help design your own nutritional programme.

Depending on how posh the Bodystat is, it will give you the following information about your Adonis-like physique:

● Body fat percentage and fat weight (often in kilograms and a scary stat to be faced with)
● Lean mass percentage and body lean mass (or muscle mass percentage)
● Total weight
● Body water percentage
● Basal metabolic rate – very similar to resting metabolic rate
● Body mass index
● Waist/hip ratio
● Average daily calorie requirement for your level of activity

Although not as accurate as lab testing, these little machines are getting better all the time and will give you a very good idea how much energy you burn off at rest. You have the chance to do the maths and work out to a reasonably high level of accuracy how much of your diet should consist of carbohydrates.

It's all very well sports nutrition books telling you that as an active sportsman your diet should consist of around 60 per cent carbohydrate, but from the result obtained from the Bodystat, you can work out how grams you need per day to achieve optimal performance – without the worry that you are eating too much or too little.

STEP TWO: GET OUT YOUR CALCULATOR

So you've had an electrical current pass through your body and you know with a certain degree of accuracy how many calories you burn off every day while taking into account your activity levels.

Of course, without a sports scientist putting you through your paces on a treadmill, you will not have an accurate figure of how much energy you expend when you run but the information you have from the Bodystat will be there – or thereabouts.

For argument's sake, let's say that based on your height, weight, age, gender and activity levels the Bodystat has come back with an average daily calorie requirement for your level of activity of 3000 calories.

Based on the general estimation that 60 per cent of an active sportsman's diet should consist of carbohydrate, you should be looking to consume 1800 calories of carbohydrate every day to give you the correct energy balance to meet exercise and training demands, fuel your own physiological metabolism to keep your organs functioning. At the same time you will avoid overeating and the danger of growing those unwanted love handles.

To put all this in simple terms: 1 gram of carbohydrate gives you 4 calories of energy.

So, to save you the maths: 1800 calories = 450 grams of carbs.

This method of working out your daily carbohydrate requirements is still not as accurate as that employed by Premiership players – but it is still one hell of a lot more accurate than taking a wild stab in the dark.

With this information at your disposal you can go into training and, more importantly, a match with the peace of mind that you have not only the right fuel in the form of carbohydrate but also the right amount of fuel in the tank to go the whole 90 minutes and leave your less nutritionally-minded opponents for dead.

ADVANCED CARBOHYDRATE NUTRITION:
THE GLYCAEMIC INDEX

After a little hesitation, I have decided to give you a little bit of advanced information on the benefits of choosing certain types of carbohydrates which are either high or low on the glycaemic index (GI).

The theory behind the GI was first put forward and developed by Dr David Jenkins in an effort to help diabetics stabilise their blood sugar levels. But not only are the principles essential for diabetics, but runners can also benefit from having a better understanding and help them choose the correct types of carbohydrates at certain times of the day.

Put simply, the GI measures the magnitude of the blood sugar response to different foods. Whenever we eat, our body has an insulin response to each type of food – in this case the varying types of carbohydrate.

When we eat meat our insulin response is minimal. Meat contains negligible amounts of carbohydrate. Glucose, however – the simplest form of carbohydrate – provokes a large insulin response. The GI is based on the body's response to glucose and all foods are compared to it. On the GI, glucose has a rating of 100. It's the food which makes the body secrete the largest amount of insulin.

The GI response to carbohydrate-rich foods is heavily influenced by what other food is eaten in conjunction.

The insulin response to a bowl of white pasta (GI of 72) eaten with a creamy and meaty sauce will not be as great as it would be if you had eaten the pasta on its own – other hormones have a direct affect on the amount of insulin secreted.

Below are examples of common high and low GI foods:

HIGH GLYCAEMIC FOODS 60–100

Bread		Cereals		Fruit	
dark rye	76	cornflakes	83	watermelon	72
white wheat	72	shredded wheat	69	pineapple	65
whole wheat	69	Rice Krispies	82	banana	60
corn meal	68	Swiss muesli	60	raisins	60

Baked goods		Grain		Vegetables	
rice cakes	92	white rice	92	baked potato	83
doughnut	76	cous cous	65	mashed potato	75
croissant	67	corn meal	68	carrots	74

Sugars	
glucose	100
honey	68

LOW GI FOOD – BELOW 60 PER CENT

Bread		Cereals		Fruits	
pitta	57	Special K	54	mango	55
wholemeal pitta	55	All Bran	44	grapes	46
whole rye	52	rice bran	20	orange	43
pumpernickel	49	porridge oats	49	apple	36
				grapefruit	23
				pear	36
				strawberry	32
				peach	42
				plum	24

Baked Goods		Grains	
danish	59	brown rice	57
bran muffin	59	whole rye	34
banana cake	50	noodles	48

Vegetables		Legumes		Beverages	
tomato	38	baked beans	48	orange juice	57
cucumber	24	green beans	30	pineapple	46
green peas	48	kidney beans	27	milk	28

VERY LOW GI

broccoli, cauliflower, coffee, cabbage

THE GI AND THE ENDURANCE FOOTBALLER

It isn't easy to apply the principles of the GI to you as a footballer and to understand the way that choosing different types of carbohydrate both high and low on the GI can affect your energy levels. But though the process is fairly complex it is possible – if you take your time in learning how to do it.

Put simply, foods high on the glycaemic index should be avoided by less active people in order to avoid weight gain and to maintain a constant blood sugar level. Consuming high GI foods is beneficial for those who exercise regularly and want to help maximise glycogen storage after a training session or match. This is due to the body's demands for the speedy replenishing of its carbohydrate stores.

Foods high in the GI are absorbed much more quickly into the bloodstream, helping to restock glycogen lost during training or a match. Having a banana, a glucose-rich energy drink or some other snack high in the GI is a fantastic way to reintroduce lost carbohydrate immediately after a hard session.

Ideal high GI post-exercise foods:

- A few pieces of fruit, preferably high in GI
- A slice of bread or toast with jam or honey
- An energy bar high in carbohydrate

To go into more detail about this complicated subject is beyond the boundaries of this book. All you really need to know is the basics which I have covered and if you want to delve deeper into the subject there is a large choice of books.

The diets of Premiership players will certainly contain a mixture of high, medium and low GI foods to be taken at different times of the day, so if you really want to emulate what they eat, you can easily find out how to make your energy levels go through the roof.

A FINAL WORD

Of all the different types of food that you can eat, from lamb chops to a tub of lard, carbohydrate-rich foods are the best way of getting you the energy you need to be a Duracell bunny on the football pitch. Getting it right is so important.

Too many carbohydrates in the short term overload your internal glycogen stores and in the long term make you chubby by weighing you down and making you slower. On the other hand, take in too little carbohydrate and you will run out of energy, letting your team-mates down by being physically unable to make up the ground to perform that vital tackle or put the ball in the net.

Without the help of a nutritionist you alone are responsible for designing your own nutrition programme. Use your logic and don't be afraid to tweak it now and then.

If you like to plan in advance and get a rough idea how much carbohydrate you'll require every week you can assess how many hours of training you'll be doing and at what intensity (the harder you work, the more carbohydrate you burn). Adjust your carbohydrate intake accordingly. So if you have to take a couple of days off training for whatever reason, bear in mind that your body will require less carbohydrate and cut back a bit.

To give you a helping hand and a very rough idea as to how much pasta you should be munching every day to optimise your playing and training performance, use the table below as a guide to work out how many grams of carbohydrate you should be aiming to consume everyday for the number of hours you train, depending on your weight in kilograms:

Weight	1 hour	2 hours	3 hours
50 kg	200 grams	300 grams	400 grams
60 kg	300 grams	400 grams	500 grams
70 kg	400 grams	500 grams	600 grams
80 kg	500 grams	600 grams	700 grams

Without recruiting the help of highly qualified dieticians, you have a difficult task to get your nutrition right. Yet you now have a far better idea how to do it than most of the people you play against. Be smart with your carbs and your game could improve more than you think.

OUT-MUSCLE THE OPPOSITION WITH PROTEIN

Protein is usually associated with body-building in the world of sports nutrition but its importance to footballers should not be ignored. That is not to say that you should be looking to crack the contents of a raw egg down your throat after a nasty pre-season beasting but if you skimp on good quality sources of protein in your daily diet your recovery from training and even injuries can be compromised. It can ultimately lead you to miss training sessions or key matches. Literally translated, the word protein means 'of primary importance', which clearly indicates just how significant it is.

As you are now aware, or should be, carbohydrate plays an essential role in providing you with energy. However, a lot of people do not know that protein can also have a part in providing energy for training, especially if you are running low on carbohydrate stores.

Protein is important not only as an auxiliary source of fuel to be used alongside fat and carbohydrate but also to help rebuild muscle fibres after training and play a key role in the hormonal responses to intense training.

Just to tell you that protein is important and you must eat it is all very well, but in order for you to fully appreciate its importance and its role in helping you improve your game, it helps if you learn a little more about the basics of the make-up of protein and how its inclusion (or inadvertent exclusion) from your diet could affect you.

THE BUILDING BLOCKS OF PROTEIN

Proteins are made up of long chains of amino acids. Their specific structure and order determines their type. There are a total of around 22 amino acids, some of which can be made by the body when necessary – known as non-essential amino acids – but others, known as essential amino acids, must be taken in as part of your diet.

Leaving essential amino acids out of your diet over a long period of time can lead to symptoms of ill health, albeit in a subtle way, and diminished physical performance in training. You may find your game play can be severely impaired for no apparent reason.

Eat a well-balanced, carnivorous diet and the chances of

becoming deficient in the essential amino acids are unlikely. All meat products contain sufficient amounts. Such types of food are known as 'complete proteins'. But if you don't eat meat, complete protein can come from non-animal products such as quinoa and soya.

Incomplete proteins form all those other types of food which do not contain essential amino acids. These include vegetable, fruit and grain products. As a result, if you are a vegetarian, you should pay particularly close attention to your diet so that it contains all the necessary essential amino acids required to meet the physical demands you are asking of your body. A well-balanced vegetarian diet, with a wide variety of food products, should ensure adequate amounts of all the essential amino acids but if you are in any doubt, consult a nutritional professional.

GOOD BRICKS BUILD A GOOD BODY

You'd be forgiven for believing that the genes that make you who you are from birth remain unchanged and cannot be altered, irrespective of what you eat. To a degree this may be so but it might surprise you to learn that your genes are a product of protein and replaced regularly – essentially by the food that you eat.

Your blood, enzymes and the structure of your genes consist of the protein you have eaten over the past six months. If the sources of protein in your diet are of poor quality you will build a poor-quality body which is not going to find it easy to endure a long season. It won't give your muscles, tendons and ligaments the strength to tolerate the occasional double-footed tackle or the nasty ankle tap which might aggravate your Achilles tendon. It might sound far-fetched and those tempting chicken nuggets might suit your wallet more than a juicy fillet of tuna, but it's not the most sensible economy measure you can take.

To ensure you are providing your body with the best quality building blocks, make sure the protein in your diet is high quality rather than those cheap processed meats you find in microwave meals and fast food restaurants. Lean cuts of meat from good sources and organic meats may be more expensive but your health will be much better, and better food will have a significant effect on the longevity and quality of your football career.

HOW MUCH PROTEIN?

There are many theories on the optimum amount of protein a footballer needs to consume if they are to meet the demands of the game, but there is no need to go overboard, whether you are the country's best striker or your club's crappest sub. Leave it to professional body-builders to consume steaks weighing the same as a new-born baby and remember you are a footballer – not a power-lifter.

There is a fairly large middle ground when it comes to the amount of protein said to be optimal for athletes performing intermittent, high-intensity running over 90 minutes. However, if you fall outside the recommended levels, your performance will certainly be hindered. On one hand, taking on too little protein delays recovery and re-synthesis of working muscles; on the other, if the body takes in more protein than it can utilise, it is broken down into waste products by the liver and some of that is converted into fat.

Books on protein requirements for sportsmen each have their own range of suggested amounts but you will not go far wrong if you aim to consume somewhere in the region of 1.1-1.5 grams of protein per kilogram of bodyweight.

PREMIERSHIP SECRET

During in-depth discussions with a leading Premiership nutritionist, who naturally wishes to remain anonymous (and much to my frustration was even then still very guarded), I was fascinated to learn that in recent years the importance of protein intake for players, particularly during pre-season training, has gone up in importance. New research suggests protein requirements are significantly increased when players do intense anaerobic training. The production of lactic acid increases the need for dietary protein to help players recover from a hard session and many top clubs recommend protein intake should then be closer to 1.7 grams per kilogram of bodyweight.

One last word on protein. That big rotating slab of meat may look very tempting in the window of the kebab shop but remember it is far from being a quality piece of meat. Unless you want your muscles, tendons and ligaments to be prone to injury, steer well clear, and get your protein from choice cuts of meat and fish.

FAT

As if you didn't already know, the word 'fat' has frequently been employed over the years in terrace chants as a way of giving a bit of stick to those players who are unfortunate enough to be carrying extra weight. Managers have not escaped the ribbing either – with current Liverpool manager Rafa Benitez unfairly being informed in song format that he looks like a fat Spanish waiter.

The intake of dietary fat, however, is not necessarily consistent with being overweight and omitting it entirely from your diet, as some players I know have tried, is not a particularly smart idea.

As discussed in chapter one, carrying an extra 2-3 kilograms of fat on your body can affect your performance on the park in a big way, weighing you down and making running that much harder. If you are truly serious about improving your physical condition and want to lose some lard from your love handles, then a complete nutritional approach to your total calorie intake from carbohydrates, protein *and* fat should be evaluated.

At 9 calories per gram, fat is the most condensed form of energy you can eat and is stored in the body in abundance. The following facts about the blubber you carry on your body might surprise you – even if you consider yourself to be on the skinny side:

● A person with less than 10 per cent of total body fat still has enough to provide sufficient energy for running literally hundreds of miles

● A football player with just 12 per cent body fat weighing 65 kilograms (just over 10 stone) will carry a staggering 7.8 kilograms of subcutaneous fat (fat which is stored under the skin). It effectively provides over 70,000 calories of energy

Whichever way you look at it, fat is an incredibly valuable energy source for the body and as such it is used and stored by the body to safeguard against times of famine. Of course, in our civilised society, with its abundance of chip shops and pizza houses, we are lucky enough not to face overwhelming hunger in the UK in the near future, but our bodies have not evolved at the same rate as such wondrous inventions as deep-fat fryers and kebab houses.

SO MUCH ENERGY – SO LITTLE USE!
You'd be forgiven for wondering why the hell the body doesn't just use its own fat stores to fuel your muscles on the football pitch. Why the reliance on carbohydrates?

Due to its chemical structure and its complexity, the way it can be broken down and used to provide energy, fat is the body's preferred (though not sole) fuel source in low intensity activities such as sitting, sleeping, walking and jogging slowly, etc. Fat will be the supply store for any situation that doesn't require energy quickly, with back-up from protein and carbohydrate.

Unfortunately for you, a footballer who tears around the park like a blue-arsed fly, as energy requirements increase for activities such as running, fat is used far less than readily-usable sources such as carbohydrate.

To have a clear picture of how the body uses both fat and carbohydrate as energy sources during exercise and at rest consider these facts:

- When running at 100 per cent of your maximum effort you are burning pretty much 95 per cent carbohydrate and just 5 per cent fat
- When sitting on your butt watching Rafa Benitez go nuts on the touchline during *Match of the Day* you are using closer to 95 per cent of fat to supply the energy and just 5 per cent carbohydrate. (Note: these figures are for illustration purposes only.)

These facts often throw players (indeed, anyone interested in losing weight) into a state of confusion as they wonder why the hell we exercise to lose body fat when by sitting on your arse you can burn a higher percentage of fat to provide your body with energy. And why are top class players in the Premiership who train for several hours a day not chubby?

Answer? It's all about the percentages.

Take the player who goes for an early, pre-season, gentle 30-minute jog at about 50 per cent of his maximum effort. At this intensity, he will burn about 200 calories, 60 per cent of which come from fat. However, if he decided to walk or even sit down for 30 minutes he would burn 80 and 90 per cent of the calories from fat respectively.

Aha, but the big question is, how many calories in total is our example burning while walking or sitting down? Not that many! Even though by sitting down he is burning 90 per cent of his energy from fat stores, the total amount of energy expended is negligible. So that's 90 per cent of nothing very much.

So, he then sets out for another 30-minute run, but this time at 75 per cent of his maximum capacity. Now he's working harder and sweating like Ronaldo when he's got a hair out of place. Our example will burn closer to 400 calories, 35 per cent of which comes from fat.

Do the maths:

Low-intensity exercise – 60 per cent of 200 calories
= 120 fat calories
High-intensity exercise – 35 per cent of 400 calories
= 140 fat calories

And that's not all. After the faster-paced run, your metabolic rate remains raised for longer with the result that you burn even more calories at rest.

So, we've established that as nice as it would be, it's not easy to utilise massive amounts of your 70,000-plus calories of body fat for an energy source while playing or training; yet cutting out all forms of dietary fat altogether is not only impossible but also makes for a pretty dull and tasteless diet.

Some types of fat are hugely beneficial for your body and joints and I strongly suggest you eat them regularly. At the same time, certain other fats should be avoided as much as possible.

GOOD FAT AND BAD FAT

Although all forms of fat contain a whopping 9 calories per gram, not all fat is the same. Despite the bad press that fatty foods receive, certain types are in fact vital for good health and must therefore be included in any player's diet, whether they play for Chelsea or Cirencester FC.

Without fat we would be unable to store and utilise the fat-soluble vitamins A, D, E, F and K – which are essential for everyday bodily functions such as vision, the absorption of calcium and blood-clotting.

The different types of fat that we eat are either saturated or unsaturated fat (mono- and polyunsaturated).

SATURATED FAT

Saturated fat is bad fat – the type that dominates nearly every food you'll take on the terraces from the fast-food outlets. Pies, pasties, kebabs and fish and chips are all dripping in saturated fat and should be avoided if you aspire to improve your condition and playing performance.

Saturated fat is found in all animal products and is easily identifiable as it is solid at room temperature and invariably ends up smeared all over your face when it drips off the end of your Mega-Burger.

Although saturated fat helps to insulate us and is necessary to provide protection for our vital organs, it is generally acknowledged that a diet high in it leads to obesity, heart disease and hundreds of thousands of premature deaths every year. You may think it's only older people who need to worry about those kinds of health conditions, but worth bearing in mind that excessive fat can still cause high cholesterol even in your 30s and hinder your fitness regime. So, think twice before playing the I'm-too-young card.

Avoiding saturated fat completely is virtually impossible, but it is important to try to minimise the amount you eat. Put simply, consuming excess saturated fat can contribute to an increase in total body fat, making you heavier and less able to haul yourself around the pitch over 90 minutes. Tips for avoiding eating excess saturated fat:

- Trim off any excess fat on meat products such as lamb, pork and beef steaks
- Avoid eating the skin on poultry and game products
- Limit red meat consumption to a maximum of twice a week
- Avoid as far as possible high fat meat, fried and dairy products such as sausages, bacon, burgers, cheese, French fries, mayonnaise, butter cream and ice cream
- Drain away excess fat from cooked meats such as minced beef
- Avoid all fast food restaurants
- Instead of frying foods, try grilling them instead.

MONOUNSATURATED FAT
Now for the good news.

Monounsaturated fats are in products such as olive, nuts, seeds and avocados and are acceptable to consume in small quantities. Olive oil is perhaps the best known type of monounsaturated fat and its health benefits are widely accepted due to its positive effect on cholesterol. Monounsaturated fats have the ability to help to lower cholesterol, providing major health benefits to everyone.

Cold-pressed, extra virgin olive oil drizzled over a salad is not only delicious but incredibly good for you. An intake of moderate amounts of monounsaturated fat is acceptable for footballers, but care must be taken that you don't overdo it.

It is still fat.

POLYUNSATURATED FATS

Polyunsaturated fats are slightly more complicated, but they provide us with a number of health benefits, such as two types of essential fatty acids. Neither of these are made by the body and do have to come as part of your diet.

These essential fatty acids – omega-3 (fish oils and flax/linseed) and omega-6 (vegetable oil) should certainly feature in the diet of a player due to their ability to produce hormone-like substances known as prostaglandins. Prostaglandins carry out a number of essential physiological functions:

- Regulation of insulin release
- Regulation of moods
- Regulation of cholesterol levels
- Help in reducing inflammation (essential for injury recovery)
- Help to prevent the immune system from over-reacting
- Maintenance of water balance
- Regulation of metabolism

The function of prostaglandins is complex but, as you can see from the list above, many of the roles they play are essential to any footballers keen to function to the best of their ability.

Key points about fat in your diet:

- Try to limit your intake of saturated fat
- Eat oily fish such as salmon, herring or mackerel twice a week
- Consume olive oil from the bottle, rather than frying foods with it
- Supplement your diet with pre-prepared essential oil products. (Always seek professional advice first.)
- Get in the habit of reading food labels to see if a food has a high fat content
- Try to consume no more than 100 grams of fat a day. You should ideally be aiming for 70 grams

CHAPTER FIVE
NUTRITIONAL SUPPLEMENTS
PILLS FOR
PERFORMANCE

As the years go by and the Premiership is worth ever more, the pressure on clubs and players to deliver the goods is even more important. The need for an extra competitive edge – on top of highly scientific training regimes and individualised nutritional programmes – is essential if teams are to get one over their rivals and bring home the silverware.

As the science and research into human performance has become more detailed and accurate through new and innovative research techniques, so the quest for the perfect nutritional supplement continues. Maybe it has already been found and the limits of legal supplementation have been reached but, where there is the demand for stronger and fitter athletes, the research will continue into that elusive perfect pill which makes players faster for longer or heal quicker

Of course, as far too many world-class sprinters have

discovered, taking illegal – yet highly effective – performance-enhancing drugs is not only foolish and cheating but also a career-ending decision which ultimately wins little peer respect and even less from (former) fans.

In the Premiership, players are tested up to five times a year to ensure they are not taking illegal substances. Any hint of wrong-doing by players is taken incredibly seriously, with lengthy bans and fines the minimum punishment that can be expected.

With so much at stake and a weekly pay packet that could revive a recession, Premiership players would be out of their minds to play with the system and risk enhancing their physicality at the potential expense of their career.

As a result, legal and approved nutritional supplements, sometime referred to as ergogenic aids, are taken by virtually every player to complement their energy-boosting diets and speed-enhancing training regimes.

Many amateur and recreational players often ask me: 'What supplements do the top players take to improve their performance?', 'Can I buy them on the high street?' and 'Is there any danger in taking them?'

This chapter will tell you all you need to know about which nutritional supplements have been scientifically proven to enhance performance, which ones there is still some debate about and which ones you really shouldn't bother spending your money on.

If used correctly and in conjunction with both a good nutritional programme and a decent training regime, certain nutritional supplements really can enhance your performance on the pitch – as a high percentage of Premiership players know. If they can benefit from them then why can't you?

BUT BEFORE YOU START POPPING PILLS

The information you are about to read is cutting-edge stuff and gives you the very latest research on a range of supplements and their effect on human performance.

However, please do not abuse this research. Just because the supplements outlined below can be purchased on the high street or even in the supermarket it does not mean that you can go bonkers and double up the dose in an effort to get twice the performance-enhancing benefits. The chances are that any increased speed on the park in that situation will only be due to you running back into the changing rooms to evacuate the contents of three days of food.

Overdosing on most supplements can severely aggravate the gut so, whatever you do, stick to the recommended doses – you'll only end up embarrassed.

Another thing to remember is that although sports supplements can be tolerated and utilised by many people, some may simply not agree with your system – and you can be one of those who will suffer ill effects. Just because a mate is raving about how some supplement has improved his performance does not necessarily mean that you will benefit from it in the same way. Even if you stick to the recommended dosage there is a chance that your body might reject it and give you a range of symptoms from dizziness to the world falling out of your derriere.

Clearly, this is far from being performance-enhancing.

If you're one of the unlucky ones, don't keep popping the pills in the hope that your body will all of a sudden accept it – try a different supplement. Any decision about performance-enhancing supplements has to be taken by you and not because you feel you should or because your mate or your Premiership idol takes the same thing. If you're not comfortable putting something manufactured in a lab into your system, then don't.

Above all, do bear in mind that just because you can buy these supplements over the counter it doesn't necessarily follow that they are weak or mild. In fact, some of the following supplements are banned in some countries for use by athletes and some are restricted to just a small amount in the bloodstream during a sporting event.

Respect the potency of these supplements and if you are in any doubt about taking them or if you feel unwell or suffer any ill effects, do the smart thing and chuck them away. Your game will only suffer if you put the wrong chemicals in your body.

Now the only choice you've got to make is which supplements to buy.

With so many different names, derivatives and prices on the market it's a minefield deciding which are effective and which aren't worth the packaging they come in.

CREATINE – THE KING OF SUPPLEMENTS
No matter how little you know about ergogenic aids or food supplements, the chances are that you will have come across creatine.

Due to powerful marketing and misinformed columnists who write sensationalist articles, many people get inaccurate information about the benefits of creatine and as a result there are a lot of footballers and athletes out there who are using it wrongly. This can affect performance, to say nothing of the damage it might cause in terms of health.

Yet creatine remains one of the most popular and effective supplements you can buy over the counter to enhance physical performance. If used correctly, your speed endurance and recovery between high-intensity sprints on the pitch can really be enhanced and your opposite number will be eating your dust.

HOW DOES IT WORK?

So, to clear up any confusion, the following information is an overview about what creatine is, how it can boost your performance and how much is safe to take.

Creatine is found naturally in meat and fish and stored in our cells. This in itself dispels a common myth, that creatine is concocted in a laboratory by men in white coats.

Back in chapter one, I gave an overview of how muscles are fuelled during a game and how they require a substance known as creatine phosphate to provide them with instant and explosive energy to contract. Internal storage of creatine is limited, so the body only has 5-8 seconds worth before its supplies – and you! – are exhausted.

If explosive and maximal (or near maximal) movement continues, the body will be unable to provide working muscles with further amounts of creatine due to the simple fact that it needs time to recover. Through sheer bloody-mindedness and determination some players will try and keep going through that phase of creatine depletion but when your thighs feel like they have had liquid fire poured on them there's only so far that determination will get you until you just seize up.

So, as if you hadn't already worked it out, this depletion of internal creatine stores can be overcome, to a degree, with an artificial supplement in the form of creatine monohydrate. In high-intensity, high-power sports such as sprinting, creatine is the only substance able to replenish instant energy stores fast enough to maintain explosive movement. That's why creatine supplementation has become one of the most popular ergogenic aids for athletes.

Put simply, by increasing the amount of creatine in the body, not only can explosive bouts of exercise can be maintained for longer and dramatic improvements made in recovery time, but you will be more resistant to fatigue. It won't make you run faster, but you will be able to maintain that pace for longer.

THE EVIDENCE FOR CREATINE

Those who believe everything they see in a book will no longer be reading this. They will already have flung it across the room and be halfway into town to pick up the biggest and most colourful tub of creatine they can find in preparation to supercharge their thighs for the next fixture.

The more cynical among you will need solid evidence that creatine is effective in improving your performance. Read on.

Since its surge in popularity after the Barcelona Olympics in 1992, when several British sprinters gave testimonials about its performance-enhancing effects, creatine's popularity has continued to rocket, as athletes in high intensity sports from football to rugby started experimenting. Scientists even got into the act and got all excited about how effective it was in improving explosive exercise. Some even dubbed creatine a legal steroid. Although many boffins would now view this claim as a little fanciful, it nevertheless shows the impact on performance enhancement that creatine had in the early '90s.

Creatine-frenzied scientists have calmed down a little in the years since then. Detailed research has been undertaken to see just how effective it is, if at all, and if there are any side effects which could cause damage to internal filtering organs such as the liver and kidneys.

I could spend the rest of this book detailing all the studies which have been done, but to summarise I will tell you that the overwhelming body of evidence stacks in favour of creatine being a highly effective supplement for boosting performance. The general consensus is that taking it in that form has the following effects on performance:

● Increases the re-synthesis/regeneration of creatine stores within the muscles between bouts of high intensity work
● Makes more creatine (therefore more readily-available energy) for subsequent bouts of high intensity work – such as sprinting for the ball
● Enhances the performance of repeated 6-30 second

bouts of maximal exercise interspersed with short periods of recovery (20 seconds to three minutes) – ideal conditions for footballers

The French Agency of Medical Security for Food asserts that the use of creatine supplements is 'against the spirit of sportsmanship and fair competition'. If that isn't enough to prove that creatine is arguably the most kick-arse supplement you can take to skin anyone you play against, laboratory tests carried out on athletes showed that loading the body with creatine does indeed enhance performance.

The results of just some of these trials are shown in the table below:

Event	Subject	Creatine dose	Results
Running 4 x 300 metres with 4 minute rest and 4 x 1 kilometre with 3 minute rest	10 trained middle distanced runners	30 grams a day for 6 days	Improved performance by reducing running time in final 300 metres and 1 kilometre runs
Jumping and running 5 seconds and 45 seconds continuous jumping exercises. Treadmill running at 20 kilometres an hour to exhaustion.	8 sprinters and 6 male jumpers	20 grams a day for 5 days	Improved jumping performance in the first and second 15 second period of jumping test and improved running time to exhaustion
Running 2 x treadmill sprints to exhaustion	11 male interval and strength-trained subjects	20 grams a day for 4 days and 10 grams a day for 6 days	Time to exhaustion improved and running times to exhaustion improved more in second run

Table adapted from Clinical Sports Nutrition *by Vicki Deakin and Louise Burke, McGraw-Hill, 2002*

Many other trials have been carried out by various laboratories to determine the effectiveness of creatine. Some trials have proved less positively conclusive than others but the vast majority – those involving tests in which subjects were given a short recovery time – proved that creatine has a positive effect on performance.

There is the evidence. Now all you've got to decide is whether you want to take it. Like any supplement, everyone's internal body chemistry handles creatine differently and some may experience side effects.

SIDE EFFECTS OF CREATINE SUPPLEMENTATION

On a personal level, I have tried to supplement my training with creatine a number of times over the years and I have never got on with it particularly well. I experienced some of the most common side effects, which include:

- Nausea
- Gastrointestinal upsets
- Dizziness
- Headaches
- Muscle cramps

Obviously, there is some room for argument that I shouldn't have been such a girl and instead of whinging about the side effects I should have persevered with bad guts and headaches if it meant improving my athletic performance. This is the trap many athletes fall into with all kinds of supplements and it's so important that you apply logic if you start feeling adverse effects.

Some indeed can be temporary and are easily overcome with a healthy dose of manliness. But it's different if they are persistent and end up negatively affecting your performance during training or a game. You've got to question why you are taking anything that really isn't helping. It is there to enhance your speed endurance and improve your recovery time between sprints, so what is the point in taking it if you're playing through a splitting headache and you feel like the world is about to fall out of your arse?

CONCLUSION

Many clubs and players keep their exact nutritional and supplemental secrets very close to their chest but you can bet your grandma that a very high percentage in the Premiership will take creatine regularly to improve their athleticism and fitness levels. But it is a potent supplement. Just because you can buy it in the same store that sells vitamin pills, don't assume you can take double doses without suffering the consequences.

And even in the Premiership, there will be a selection of players whose systems just can't tolerate it and will have no choice but to leave it well alone. Creatine is probably one of the most effective supplements you can take but only if your system likes it. Do not be afraid to bin it if you suffer from side effects.

The sale of creatine is banned in France with some studies hinting that it might be carcinogenic. Others indicate that long-term use could lead to kidney damage. The (long term) use of creatine is not to be embarked upon lightly. By all means take it – it is totally legal in the UK and the USA – but always exercise caution. Enjoy opening an almighty can of whoop-ass on your opponents and leave them for dead. But if your guts are telling you that they don't get on with it, listen to them.

COFFEE FOR PERFORMANCE

The notion that you could use caffeine to improve athletic performance was once laughed at by experts and athletes alike, but now there is a stack of scientific data to support the claim that it is a significant performance-enhancing drug.

It is not on the list of banned substances today, but until 2004 Olympic athletes were only allowed a certain amount of caffeine in their bloodstream and higher levels were considered to be a 'deliberate attempt to gain an advantage'. Amounts are still closely monitored by the World Anti-Doping Agency even today. Should higher levels feature consistently in successful athletes there is every chance that the ban will be reintroduced.

How can a cup of coffee make you a better athlete and footballer? Can a Starbucks grande latte an hour before kick-off really give you the energy you need to express physical dominance on the park?

Not really. You'd need more than the average mug to see any improvements in your performance. But caffeine really can give you the boost that your game might just need if it's taken properly. The secret is in knowing how to take it, when to take it, *where* to take it (this last will bring tears to the eyes when I explain it later) and how much to take. If you get any of these elements wrong caffeine will be utterly useless. It's essential you get the supplement guidelines right to get the maximum effect from the world's most popular, powerful and legal drug.

HOW DOES IT WORK?

Caffeine is a central nervous system stimulant – that's why it is used by millions of people every morning to give themselves a kick up the arse when they get out of bed.

Like amphetamines, caffeine improves alertness, concentration, reaction time and energy levels – the very functions that any footballer could do with sharpening to gain an advantage on the field.

Caffeine directly affects the central nervous system in the following ways:

- Increasing mental alertness
- Increasing concentration
- Decreasing fatigue and delaying the onset of fatigue
- Increasing reaction time
- Increasing the use of muscle triglyceride (making you burn more fat)

Without doubt, the physiological effect that caffeine has on the body has a lot to offer you in the way of giving you that extra competitive edge during a game, but knowing exactly how to use it is essential.

HOW MUCH CAFFEINE DO YOU NEED TO ENHANCE PERFORMANCE?

As with creatine, dozens of studies have been conducted into discovering the ideal amount of caffeine required to boost performance and endurance.

Although each trial tests different variables, there is now overwhelming evidence that sufficient amounts of caffeine prior to exercise can make you a better athlete. The trouble is that the amount of caffeine you need to give you these mind-blowing improvements in athletic ability is quite a bit more than you'd find in an average cup – even with an extra shot! To give you an idea just how much caffeine is need to make it ergogenic, consider the approximate caffeine content of the following beverages.

Strong cup of tea	80-90 milligrams of caffeine
Cup of instant coffee	50-60 milligrams of caffeine
Cup of very strong-brewed coffee	130-150 milligrams of caffeine
Can of Red Bull	80 milligrams of caffeine
Can of Coke	50 milligrams of caffeine
Double espresso	100 milligrams of caffeine
Grande latte	150 milligrams of caffeine

These figures will of course vary according to the type of drink and the size of the cup, but you're looking at a maximum of 180 milligrams of caffeine per cup of very strong coffee. That's what will be coursing through your veins just before kick-off – and will it turn you into a supercharged football machine? Well, not really. I'm afraid 180 milligrams just doesn't quite cut the mustard.

Studies have shown that you should aim to be taking something like twice that amount, though the amount will vary as some people are much more (or less) responsive. But broadly speaking, scientists suggest you should be aiming to consume somewhere in the region of 5 milligrams of caffeine per kilogram of body weight.

Let's consider that you are a 70kg player:

milligrams of caffeine x 70 kilograms = 350 milligrams of caffeine

To put that figure into perspective, you might look at getting that boost from:

- Two Starbucks grande lattes
- More than three double espressos
- Four cans of Red Bull
- Seven cans of Coke

However, it's interesting to see the selection of studies in *Clinical Sports Nutrition* by leading dieticians Louise Burke and Vicki Deakin. Their book is widely considered to be the sports nutrition bible and it shows that huge doses of caffeine are not always necessary to gain a competitive edge.

Due to variations in an athlete's physiological response to caffeine and training intensities, performance improvements have been seen anywhere from 3 milligrams per kilograms up to a massive 10 milligrams per kilogram (that's seven double espressos or nine cans of Red Bull).

The following table highlights three studies conducted to test athletes running at a similar intensity to that of a footballer. It measures the effect of different amounts of caffeine on performance.

Event	Subjects	Caffeine	Results
Running at 85 per cent VO2 max	9 well-conditioned male athletes	4.5 milligrams per kilogram	Increased time to exhaustion
Running at 85 per cent VO2 max	8 trained men	3,6,9 milligrams per kilogram	Improved running performance seen with the 3 and 6 milligrams per kilogram dose
Running 75 per cent VO2 Mmax then incremental to exhaustion	6 recreational male runners	10 milligrams per kilogram immediately before exercise	Caffeine increased total distance run

Table adapted from Clinical Sports Nutrition by Vicki Deakin and Louise Burke, McGraw-Hill, 2002

All subjects demonstrated performance benefits from taking caffeine with doses ranging from 3 milligrams per kilogram to 10 milligrams per kilogram. On the face of it this should be encouraging for you as a recreational footballer. There is of course a 'but'.

Knowing the amount of caffeine you need to get into your system is one thing, but you also need to know the best way to do it without making yourself violently ill.

HOW, WHEN AND WHERE TO TAKE CAFFEINE
It wasn't so long ago that a hundred random people asked in true *Family Fortunes* style to name the country's most popular caffeinated drink would probably come up with coffee as the top answer. Tea and Coke would be very close behind.

But in recent years the surge in popularity of the highly caffeinated Red Bull would perhaps match coffee in popularity. Given the ease with which it can be knocked back prior to a game, Red Bull now stands as one of the most popular drinks that recreational runners and players use before an event or game to get their caffeine fixed and body buzzed for the task ahead.

In the same way, highly potent caffeine tablets have also gained in popularity. You can get the maximum caffeine boost out of them but without surplus liquid sloshing around your stomach as you chase down your opponent.

I mentioned at the beginning of the caffeine section that I would explain *where* caffeine can also be taken to enhance performance. As ambiguous and intriguing a concept as this sounds, I can tell you now it is not for the faint-hearted. Not to be recommended or advised if you're bothered by the likely reaction of sheer disgust from your team-mates.

Some top flight athletes and maybe even Premiership players – though I have yet to get a personal confession from anyone – take caffeine supplements to the next level and bypass the stomach altogether as a means to get caffeine into their system. If you remember a little of your school biology lessons, you'll already know that there is one part of the body which is surprisingly absorbent. Top sportsmen, wanting the cutting edges of cutting edges, insert their caffeine supplement in this handy cavity to maximise its benefit.

If you haven't already worked it out, I'll spell it out for you. Caffeine suppositories are used widely by athletes to get their physiological advantage. Yes, my friends, coffee and Red Bull are for girls – you want to get a caffeine boost, then shove a specially-formulated caffeine suppository up where the sun don't shine and get that caffeine into you like a real man! It's your choice of course, but personally I wouldn't recommend such an extreme method.

And whichever way footballers choose to ingest caffeine for performance-enhancing benefits, there are many potential problems which can be experienced.

SIDE EFFECTS OF CAFFEINE

There are a number of potential problems with the use of caffeine to aid your sportsmanship. As with creatine, there will always be some people who either do not respond to its ergogenic properties or suffer adverse effects. So before you go ahead and start ingesting it, bear in mind the following:

- Caffeine, like alcohol, has a diuretic effect on the body – something to bear in mind if you take it, as recommended, up to just an hour before kick-off
- Irrespective of the benefits that caffeine can provide, it must not be at the expense of water or a sports drink. If you just have coffee you may start a game dehydrated and your performance may suffer
- Excessive amounts of coffee – whether from espressos, lattes or other sources – can cause gastrointestinal discomfort. Never take large doses before a game without trailing it in practice. Mid-match gut-churn is a problem which cannot be strapped or fixed with a wet sponge
- Coffee interferes with the absorption of iron. If you are a regular coffee drinker make sure you consume iron-rich foods at a different time to your coffee intake

CONCLUSION

The fact that the World Anti-Doping Agency once banned and still has question marks over the use of caffeine in sport is an indication that caffeine may well provide significant benefits for anyone who partakes in high intensity sports such as football.

The decision to use caffeine as an ergogenic aid is not one to be taken lightly. Migraines, anxiety and nervousness are just a few of the symptoms that can result from having excessive levels of the substance in your system. If you go ahead, experiment with caffeine supplements during training sessions and always begin by taking low doses and only then working up if necessary. Use extreme caution before dosing with higher levels of caffeine. Its effects can really knock you for six and in some people cardiac health has even been compromised, sometimes seriously and permanently, by taking too much.

Remember, just because you can buy caffeine-based products anywhere on the street, from the supermarket to a service station, respect that fact that you're still taking a drug and in some cases it does not agree with some people – even in small doses. Never take it in high doses just because everyone else is. You are an individual so use your common sense and use it responsibly.

If in doubt, read more about the effects of caffeine consumption and if necessary consult your doctor.

L-CARNITINE

L-carnitine as a supplement has steadily become more popular with recreational athletes over the years. It boosts performance and many people swear by it, though there are still quite a few sports nutritionists who remain dubious about its ergogenic properties.

HOW DOES IT WORK?

L-carnitine is a naturally occurring amino acid found mainly in meat products. It is an essential nutrient for forming the transport system responsible for taking fat to the mitochondria to be burned and used as fuel. Without going into too much detail, the mitochondria are the area of your cells which is responsible for producing energy. The theory is that increasing the amount of carnitine in your body will help you to shift more fat to utilise as an energy source.

This transport system is unable to work effectively without sufficient amounts of carnitine and that leads to a reduction in the fat available to provide energy. Some sportsmen (and their nutritionists) believe that in order to boost fat oxidation (to use your stored blubber more effectively as an energy source) you need to pop a few carnitine pills. You would then be a fat-burning machine on the pitch, not only with more energy to chase down opponents but also more cut in the process.

The big question is – does it work?

Does supplementing your diet with some hardcore carnitine pills turn your fat transport system into the equivalent of a ten-lane motorway? Will your body burn off fat quicker than a Formula One car burns petrol?

WHAT IS THE EVIDENCE?

The scientific evidence of carnitine's properties is varied and – unhelpfully – mostly contradictory.

One of the world's most eminent sports nutritionists, Dr Michael Colgan, praised carnitine in his book *Optimum Sports Nutrition* (Advanced Research Press, 1999). He gave the results of trials which had taken place in 1990 involving cyclists taking two grams of carnitine. The finding was that it vastly helped in improving performance and reducing the waste products of lactate – ideal results for any footballer wanting to keep going for longer. However, more recent studies have questioned these findings and have not found any evidence that carnitine helps to utilise more fat as an energy source or that it boosts performance.

Like so many studies of nutritional supplements, those investigating the evidence for the ergogenic properties of carnitine are varied. The results leave you, the player, no better informed as to whether it is worth taking or not.

CONCLUSION

Due to the fact that there is very little strong evidence to support the claim that Carnitine boosts the oxidation of fat during exercise I'd be cautious about using it as a supplement. You can pay a small fortune for Carnitine supplements, so I'd suggest you save your money and spend it on a more effective and proven supplement.

CHAPTER SIX
FLUIDS
DRINKING FOR PERFORMANCE

In the quarter finals of the 1962 World Cup, hosts Chile figured they needed to adapt their own idea of optimum fluid replacement in order to beat strong favourites the USSR. Their idea of a sports drink punched a little bit more of a kick than those we are familiar with today. Each player knocked back a couple of vodkas and took the pitch ready to do battle.

The result?

Chile won 2-1 and progressed to the semis to face Brazil. Sadly, they chose not to follow the same pre-match drinking ritual, swapping vodka for coffee. It turned out to be a costly mistake. Brazil thrashed the hosts 4-2.

I'm sure there's a moral to that story...

The views of how and what to drink for optimum performance have, unsurprisingly, changed dramatically since

1962. The science behind the correct consumption of fluids – from coffee to water to sports drinks (to vodka) – has given players and their nutritionists the knowledge of what is best to drink before, during and after matches and what drinks are best to avoid altogether. Though the 11 players who represented Chile in that famous game against the USSR would disagree, vodka does not feature on the list of recommended beverages to consume before a game – or at all.

Fluid can be taken in a variety of ways and they all have their place in a footballer's diet. Their importance to the physical ability to play 90 minutes at near maximal intensity is right up there with carbohydrate consumption and fitness training itself.

As someone who plays recreationally, it is up to you to get your hydration right, so rather than guessing what fluids to take and at what time, you need an insight into how the pros hydrate before, during and after games and how you too can follow a similar hydration programme to play at the top of your game.

WATER

It might not ooze the same appeal as Lucozade Sport, but do not underestimate the role that plain water has in your diet.

It contains no calories and few nutrients; you'd be forgiven for wondering why water is so essential for your physical performance on the park. What it has got over a nutrient-rich pint of Guinness, bursting with B vitamins, iron and enough carbohydrate to make you run a mile?

Water is the most important substance in sustaining life,

excluding oxygen. Without water our essential organs would not be able to function properly and blood would not be pumped around the body. Just a 10 per cent decrease in our body weight through water loss can lead to death. To put this into perspective, we can afford a 40 per cent reduction in our body weight of fat, protein and carbohydrate and still survive.

As a football player putting yourself through a rigorous 90-minute workout it is essential that you keep yourself hydrated throughout the game, particularly on warm days. Avoid any drop in hydration and the risk of reduced performance that goes with it.

Staying hydrated is an essential part of training and playing in the Premiership and the nutritionists go crazy if their players do not take it seriously. They can suffer serious performance lulls when carbohydrate levels are low, but a player in a state of dehydration can really start to dwindle and may cost his team the game – even if the level of hydration drops by just 2 per cent.

If you thought the most important part of performance enhancement was loading up with carbohydrates and taking creatine and caffeine supplements – think again.

Here are a few facts about hydration to illustrate just how essential water and other fluids are for footballers – regardless of ability:

● The human body consists of around 60-70 per cent water
● Of our total daily intake of fluid, 60 per cent comes

from water, 30 per cent from food and 10 per cent from the metabolic reactions within our body

- During intense exercise performed in warm conditions over 90 minutes it is not uncommon for the body to lose 5-7 per cent of body water content, even if you take on fluids during the game
- Just a 2 per cent drop in hydration status leads to a significant rise in heart rate and core body temperature
- A 5 per cent drop in hydration status can lead to a 30 per cent reduction in prolonged aerobic capacity
- The muscles of a player's legs during a game can produce as much as 250-350 millilitres of fluid in as little as 90 minutes

If you want to give yourself any chance of matching the Premiership boys in terms of (relative) physical performance, take your fluids seriously and follow the tips in this chapter to ensure you start training and matches well watered – and ready to kick some ass!

HYDRATED OR DEHYDRATED – HOW CAN YOU TELL?

Carbohydrate depletion can make you feel a little dizzy, heavy-legged and disorientated, but the early, telltale signs of dehydration are not always immediately obvious. Thirst is often the most common sign that you need to take on fluids, but for an athlete this automatic signal from your brain to quench your thirst comes far too late. Your muscles will already be dehydrated and will not be able to function at maximum potential – and that's just the beginning.

Hydration is not easy, no matter how good a player you are. Drink too little and you begin a game dehydrated and lacking your competitive edge. Drink too much and the fluids sloshing around your stomach will give you cramps closely followed by an insatiable desire to pee like a race horse – not ideal when you are only ten minutes into the match.

As with every other aspect of physical and nutritional preparation, the cream of the Premiership are assessed individually and told what to drink, how much to drink and when to drink it. Sadly, the only time you are likely to get such strict terms are on a stag weekend and that is hardly what I'd call performance-enhancing hydration – on more than one level!

As I mentioned when discussing taking nutritional supplements, experiments with the timing and quantity of your fluid intake should be done pre-season so you know how much fluid you need to take on without putting excessive pressure on your bladder.

The best way to tell if you are properly hydrated is fairly crude but actually pretty easy if you are a bloke. All you've got to do is simply check out the colour of your urine. If you are adequately hydrated, your urine should be either clear or of a light straw colour; if you are dehydrated your urine has a stronger odour and is a deeper yellow colour. Bear in mind that if you are taking a multivitamin tablet, a high dosage of vitamin B2 can turn your urine a bright yellow colour which does not necessarily indicate dehydration.

WHAT IS YOUR RATE OF FLUID LOSS?

Okay, so you now know how to tell when you are dehydrated and that you should never set foot on the training ground or match pitch with dark yellow urine. The trouble is that it's not easy to get your hydration status spot on, especially when you don't know the rate at which you lose fluid.

Irrespective of whether you are being beasted in pre-season or you are 30 minutes into a full-on match with the temperature in the mid 20s, it is impossible to guess how much fluid you are losing through sweat. Everyone sweats at different rates. Premiership players playing early on in the season when the weather can still be very warm have been noted to lose up to a massive 2-3 litres of sweat per hour and this figure varies massively depending on the weight of each player, how much muscle mass they have and the position they play, etc.

The same physiological process applies whether you play in lower leagues or part-time in the odd five-a-side match at your local leisure centre. You have to work out what your rate of fluid loss is for your body type, the intensity that you play and your position.

You may have noticed during pre-season training sessions your rate of perspiration may not be the same as your team-mates, even though they may be blowing out of their asses as much as you. As a result, it is essential that you find out early on in your training how much fluid you lose during a hard session so that you can take steps to reduce a significant drop in hydration status.

The easiest way to give you an idea of your rate fluid loss during a match is by simply using a set of bathroom scales.

THE BATHROOM SCALES DEHYDRATION TEST

The best time to test your dehydration is during pre-season, where you will be running at similar intensities as you would be in a hard match.

Make sure you are well hydrated. Immediately before you start training and after you have taken your last pee, step on some bathroom scales and jot down your exact weight. Remember that 1 pint of water weighs 1 pound. As soon as you return from your training session – before you visit the bathroom or re-hydrate – step back on the scales and mark down your weight again. If you have had fluids during training, it is important to note how much and take that into account when you weigh yourself.

Your rate of fluid loss during training will vary enormously depending on the length of the session, how hard you have trained, the ambient temperature and humidity. Although some of your weight loss will have come from lost glycogen and fat stores, the majority will be a result of fluid loss through respiration and perspiration.

For those of you who are interested in research into the physiological adaption and effects of exercise on the active body, you'll be interested to learn that studies referenced by William Costill and Jack Wilmore indicate that a 70 kilogram football player will metabolise around 245 grams of carbohydrate and lose as much as 1500 millilitres of fluid during a one-hour run, with this figure rising in warm conditions. This fluid and carbohydrate loss can equate to a weight loss of as much as 2 kilograms.

If you want to get a really accurate idea of the rate at which you lose fluid during a match, try repeating the procedure of weighing yourself before and after training (and even after the first few matches of the season) to get a better idea of how much fluid you'll need to replace during a game to stay optimally hydrated.

By writing down your rate of fluid loss after training sessions of varying length, intensity and climate, you will be far better placed to know how much fluid you should be taking on during a match, whatever the conditions. The result will be that you will become a well-hydrated player, giving you that extra edge over dehydrated and flailing opponents in the final quarter of the match.

TIPS FOR MEASURING FLUID LOSS

Always use the same scales in the same location to ensure accurate readings:

- Make a diary of your post-training weight loss
- If you drink fluid during a match or training, take its weight into account
- Find out the expected conditions on match day and refer back to your diary to see how much fluid you can expect to lose by comparing it to previous training sessions or matches in similar conditions
- Once you have a rough idea of the amount of fluid you have lost, replace it as soon as possible. Again, remember that 1 pint (560 millilitres) in volume equals 1 pound (450 grams) in weight

THE EFFECTS OF DEHYDRATION

It is often very difficult to tell if you are dehydrated during a game. Checking the colour of your urine stream is easy to do in the changing room but during a match it's hardly practical to step up to corner flag to perform said analysis. Therefore, you have to take every step possible to ensure you remain well-hydrated using the tips explained previously.

Premiership players have certainly been trained to know the real deal about the importance of dehydration and are made to drink whenever they can to maintain high hydration status. You will have to discipline yourself on the timing and quantity of your fluid intake. If you misjudge it and slowly start to become dehydrated during a game a number of physiological processes will slowly start to have a detrimental effect on your performance and make you a weak link in the team.

It's all very well me telling you this, but to further incentivise you to take your hydration as seriously as those in the Premiership do, it's worth explaining exactly how a drop in hydration status can affect your performance. By developing an understanding into the effect dehydration has on your working leg muscles and internal organs you will be far better informed on the importance of replacing lost fluids. This will hopefully prevent you making the same schoolboy errors that your opponents may have made with their own fluids.

DON'T LET YOUR BLOOD RUN DRY

Perhaps the most significant impact of denying your body sufficient amounts of fluid is that your blood thickens into more of a gooey substance.

When you are properly hydrated, the water content of your blood plasma is around 90 per cent. This high water content ensures that the blood flows freely around the body via your arteries and capillaries, just as water flows out of a hose. The movement allows the blood to deliver essential nutrients to the working muscles so that they can continue to respond to the dynamic instructions you brain is giving them – i.e. to leg it after the ball or the shins of that cocky centre forward.

However, when you become dehydrated through excessive sweat loss and increased respiration over the course of a match, the blood becomes more viscous than watery and therefore it becomes far harder for the heart to work at its pumping duties.

This is where it starts to matter to you as the footballer. This thicker blood puts the heart under one hell of a lot more stress in order to transport essential oxygen and nutrients to fuel your thighs on the pitch. Think of the analogy about water flowing out of a hose – well, if that water was instead some kind of thick soup it wouldn't be anywhere near as effective.

For those who have other conditions – the unfit, overweight or the older – this extra stress on the heart might even be fatal but for a (reasonably) fit footballer the consequences are far less extreme. But you can still find your performance impaired and will feel utterly shattered.

Reducing the water content of your blood ultimately causes an increase in heart rate to ensure the required levels of oxygen and nutrients in the blood reach the working muscles. You might be able to tolerate this increased effort for a while and still be able to perform well on the pitch but your heart rate for even the shortest of sprints will shoot up and remain high even when you are taking a breather. This will prematurely tire you out and make that run down the touchline or chase back a far more daunting physical task than it should be.

And all this can happen as a simple result of failing to hydrate yourself properly.

The good news is that it's avoidable. The pros have known this for years and that's why they have the riot act thrown at them if they fail to take on sufficient fluids. Now you know the secret, it's time you took your fluid intake to the next level and make sure your blood is not running dry.

As a rough guide, you should be aiming to drink the following quantities of fluid before and during a match:

- 400-600 millilitres two hours before training or playing a match
- 150-300 millilitres in the last 20 minutes before a game (or 6 millilitres per kilogram of body weight)
- 150-250 millilitres every 15-20 minutes during the match if possible. On warm days you should aim for at least 250 millilitres every 15-20 minutes.

There is one question, though, which is still left unanswered. What is the best fluid to hydrate with – good old fashioned water or sports drinks like Lucozade?

WATER VS SPORTS DRINKS

There has been a lot of confusion and controversy over the years as to the genuine performance-enhancing role that sports drinks have on players. Does a bottle of Lucozade at half-time genuinely buy you that 800th or so of a second of increased energy in the dying minutes of the game? Will it give you an advantage over your opponent who's just drunk boring old water or is it all just good, old-fashioned marketing hype?

The drink of choice up and down the country is without doubt anything with 'Sports' on the side. They taste good, they look sexy and they're packed with colouring, flavouring and E-numbers. All of which makes them far more appealing than dull H_2o – yet most players don't actually have a clue if they have any significant benefits.

Well, let me tell me you that the type of fluid you drink in the lead-up, during and after a ball-busting and sweaty 90-minute game can make a significant impact on your hydration status and your general physical performance. Water may very well be the most natural of the two substances and make up over 60 per cent of your total body weight, but the rise in popularity of sports drinks over the years has not just been because of powerful marketing.

A number of scientific studies carried out on the effectiveness of isotonic sports drinks have demonstrated that they do have an advantage over water in rehydrating the body quicker and replacing lost sugars and salts. Although sports drinks should not be used as your sole source of hydration, they do play a role in helping maintain performance by ensuring the body has enough sugar and electrolytes to keep going.

It's hard to imagine, but decades ago Lucozade was not a drink that was affiliated with improving athletic performance – far from it! After initially being marketed as an essential drink for the elderly to replace lost sugars, etc, after illness, its directors made a u-turn and marketed the product to athletes. They tried to get the message across that the importance of a beverage rich in glucose and electrolytes could play a key role in enhancing performance by keeping you going for longer.

Many believed it was simply a marketing ploy but research over the years has proven that sports drinks such as Lucozade and Gatorade play a vital role in maintaining not only hydration status but also topping up the blood with sugar and electrolytes – the loss of which we now know can have a massively detrimental effect on performance and health.

SPORTS DRINKS AND SPORTS DRINKS

Although they all look pretty much the same on the outside, there are a variety of sports drinks available to players, each with varying amounts of glucose.

After reading about the importance of carbohydrate, many people automatically choose the drink with the highest percentage of glucose to help maintain blood sugar levels. The truth is a little more complicated than that due to the sensitivity of a function known as 'gastric emptying'.

GASTRIC EMPTYING

Whenever we eat food or drink, the contents of the stomach and gastric juices are absorbed into the duodenum. Here nutrients are absorbed into the bloodstream and delivered to the working muscles. Gastric emptying is the process of the movement of the contents of the stomach through to the duodenum. The time it takes for food to be broken down and absorbed is dependent on the type of food in the stomach.

In the case of sports drinks, the higher the glucose solution, the slower the rate of gastric emptying. A sports drink with a high sugar content consumed during exercise can take up to two hours to empty, compared to just 20 minutes for a weak sugar solution.

So, it is essential that you must ensure you choose a sports drink which has the correct amount of sugar in it.

SPORTS DRINKS TYPES
Hypotonic
● 2-3 grams of sugar per 100 millilitres
● Less concentrated than bodily fluids
● Absorbed quicker than water
● Fast re-hydration

Isotonic
● 5-7 grams of sugar per 100 millilitres
● Similar concentration to body fluids
● Absorbed at the same speed as water

Hypertonic
● 10 grams-plus of sugar per 100 millilitres
● Higher concentration than body fluids
● Slower absorption than water

EFFECTIVE HYDRATION FOR PERFORMANCE

For the quickest rate of fluid absorption and delivery of sugar to the blood stream, the sports drink must be isotonic with a 5-7 per cent sugar content. If you had to choose one type of sports drinks to best match the hydration and energy needs of a footballer, then the isotonic drink is the one.

Most sports drinks are manufactured with a variety of different sugars such as glucose, fructose, corn syrup and maltodextrin, as this is believed to be more effective. To help aid sugar absorption, the sports drink must also contain electrolytes as well as maintain adequate levels of salt in the bloodstream.

Isotonic drinks are probably the most common type of sports drink you can buy but do take a look at the label and check. As with ergogenic supplements, if you are not used to drinking sports drinks I'd strongly suggest you try them out first before you knock back your first bottle 30 minutes before a game. Although they are tolerated well by most people, some do have an adverse reaction to them so make sure your stomach can tolerate the sugary formula.

This popularity is a miraculous turnaround in the fortunes of a drink which was once given to old biddies recovering from an illness and now is proven to be highly effective and beneficial in providing hydration for top athletes. And the story does not end there.

The hydration and carbohydrate-replacement properties of Lucozade and co are clearly essential but the added electrolytes are also vital to prevent the potentially life-threatening condition known as hyponatremia.

ELECTROLYTES AND HYPONATREMIA

One of the reasons isotonic drinks are so effective is that they have a very similar composition to our body fluids, which contain glucose and electrolytes (salts).

Electrolytes include the minerals sodium, chloride, potassium and magnesium and are all secreted in varying amounts in our sweat – especially sodium and chloride. This is why our sweat tastes salty.

For any athletic event lasting an hour or more, particularly high intensity games such as football, the effects of dehydration, electrolyte loss and low blood sugar should not significantly affect the health of a player. However, if poor nutritional practices have been followed in the build-up to an intense match, there is a risk that the health of player could be severely compromised. And it's this little-known condition which is known as hyponatremia.

Although more common in long distance events such as marathons, in which the rate of sweat is much higher than in football, cases of hyponatremia do occur in a range of sporting events with varying degrees of severity – and at the worst that can include death.

WHAT CAUSES HYPONATREMIA?

Hyponatremia can occur for a number of reasons but it's perhaps most commonly found in players who take the importance in hydration a little too far.

Take the example of a player who is about to play in an important match at the beginning of the season and he knows the temperature on the pitch is going to be well into the 20s. To ensure he is well hydrated for the game he drinks water – a lot of water. He might be peeing like a race horse all morning but in his mind it's all good, because his hydration status is going to be awesome come kick-off.

As the match progresses and the heat really starts getting to him, his fluid loss through sweat and respiration is high, encouraging him to take on even more water to prevent dehydration.

Although this might stand to reason, what our friend doesn't know is that throughout the morning and during the game he is actually diluting his blood of essential salts and lowering their electrolyte content. He faces additional salt loss in the shape of sweat he is secreting through the heat on the pitch. If the drop in electrolytes becomes severe enough, it may bring on hyponatremia. Symptoms include confusion, disorientation, nausea and weakness.

Proof that sometimes a little knowledge can be a dangerous thing. Water is fantastic and essential to use to rehydrate the body but if you drink copious amounts on the days leading up to a game and dilute your internal salt stores and compound that by losing more salt by sweating like a horse in a French abattoir, you could find yourself in all kinds of trouble.

Cases of hyponatremia are rare in football but it is highly recommended that on hot days you use a bottle of sports drink or two to replace lost salts. That said, although sports drinks are used by many of the country's top players, they do not rely on it as their sole source of fluid replacement. One nutritionist I spoke to actually advises players to use them sparingly and only in certain circumstances – during hot and intense matches, for example. This particular nutritionist believes on the whole they are too sweet and in most instances water remains a better form of hydration, at least in the more regular playing conditions.

HOW TO AVOID HYPONATREMIA

- Avoid drinking excessive amounts of water on the morning of the days leading up to a match
- Take advantage of the sports drink stations during half-time
- Do not deliberately avoid salty foods in the lead up to a game but also ensure you do not consume excessive amounts.

To summarise, do not underestimate how important is to get your hydration right if you are really looking for that extra competitive edge. Whereas the golden boys of the Premiership are well looked-after and told what to drink, when to drink and how much of it they need to drink you do not have that luxury – so you're on your own.

Remember, you are an individual with your own hydration requirements and needs. Do not be tempted to drink what all your mates are drinking because you feel you should. Find out what your rate of fluid loss is during pre-season so that you know how much fluid you lose during a 90-minute game and how much you should be replacing.

Games are won by the smallest of margins and getting your hydration status right could quite easily mean the difference between kicking some ass and having some ass kicked.

CHAPTER SEVEN

MANAGE YOUR INJURIES LIKE THE PROS

THE SECRETS FOR HEALING FAST

INJURIES THAT PREMIERSHIP STARS WOULD RATHER WE DIDN'T KNOW ABOUT

Shaun Goater, Manchester City

You'd think lessons would be learned after coming a cropper once from a goal celebration, but Goater clearly still had a few problems controlling his excitement. The first time he let his excitement get the better of him was in 1998 when he scored against Stoke City. A delighted Goater jumped up, fell and broke his arm.

The second time was some five years later in 2003. In a frenzied moment of pure excitement after Anelka scored a crucial goal, Goater headed over to the sidelines and released his pent-up euphoria by kicking an advertising board a little zealously, badly damaging his knee in the process.

Alan Mullery, Tottenham Hotspur and England

There are some injuries which, although embarrassing, are very understandable. There have been plenty of occasions over the years when players have been picked up by their team-mates after scoring a winning goal and accidentally dropped to the floor, breaking a bone or two in the process. They are injuries which should not really happen and can hardly be displayed as war wounds picked up with honour in the heat of battle after a bruising encounter with a rival team. But they happen, every now and again.

Mullery sustained a back injury in 1964 which made him unable to travel with the England team to South America. But he couldn't blame his condition on his team-mates, his opponents or even a nasty fall during training or a match. Sadly, his back injury was sustained in an incident far more embarrassing than that. Although I'm sure he'd fight every step of the way for the tale not to be continually retold and eventually inscribed on his gravestone, Mullery managed to put his back out in the course of brushing his teeth. The details are unclear but all I know is that a once-in-a-lifetime opportunity to travel with his country to tour South America was thwarted by an over-enthusiastic attempt to make those shiny whites even whiter.

David Batty, Leeds, Blackburn and Newcastle

Most top-flight footballers will injury themselves on the pitch, either during a match or on the training field, so you can imagine the quizzical looks David Batty must have received from his team (information is patchy on the way his colleagues were informed) when he hobbled into the club with a nasty Achilles tendon injury. But in his case what could have been a career-threatening injury was sustained from a most unlikely source – a collision with a small child on a tricycle. Just how much abuse he copped from his teammates can only be guessed but I can't imagine he would have got away with it lightly.

INJURIES ARE ALL PART OF THE GAME

Irrespective of ability, as a footballer you have to accept the fact that at some time or other you are going to get injured.

Research has shown that the overall incidence is between 0.5 and 13 injuries per 1000 hours of football in adolescents and 9 and 35 injuries per 1000 hours of football in adults. If nothing else, the stats clearly show that there is a direct relationship between incidences of injury and the ageing player.

The same study also revealed that although the majority were minor, football players suffer a higher incidence of injury in comparison with those who participate in rugby, hockey, judo, boxing and basketball.

Like it or not, injuries are part of the game and – as frustrating as it is to be sidelined for few weeks with a sprained ankle, hamstring tweak or broken metatarsal – you've just got to man up and accept it.

Premiership players enjoy the luxury of 24-hour rehabilitation for any injury. It gives them the best chance of getting back on the pitch playing to earn their astronomical weekly wage. In direct contrast, you, as a recreational player, training just a few times a week and also having to deal with your full-time job, are likely to have at your disposal a Tubigrip, a bag of peas in the freezer and a few tubes of Deep Heat.

Injuries in part-time players are often a real source of frustration and can be stubborn in treatment, particularly if you don't have the bank balance of a Premiership footballer and have to pay for four or five sessions of physiotherapy treatment or sports massage. But don't worry too, as this chapter will give you a massive helping hand to manage your injuries better. First and foremost, you will learn how to prevent certain injuries in the first place – prevention is always better than cure. Secondly, you will gain an insight into some of the tricks and tips that physios at top clubs use to treat players. You can use them on a budget to treat your own injuries and get you back playing as soon as possible.

PREVENTION IS BETTER THAN CURE

Pre-habilitation, or the process of conditioning the body correctly to prevent certain injuries happening in the first place, is a relatively new concept in the world of football – at the top level let alone in the lower leagues. Yet in many cases conventional injuries such as hamstring tears and groin strain can be prevented. All you need is a little knowledge about your body and to learn a series of very simple exercises which you can perform before, during and after training and matches in order to protect certain structures and prevent those niggling injuries which have the potential to give you grief for months.

The two key pre-habilitation modalities Premiership players use to prevent injuries are:

● Core strength and stability
● Proprioception exercises

The good news for you is that these approaches to injury prevention and management are not part of the exclusive science that only multi-million pound clubs can afford for their treasured golden boys.

By developing an understanding of the following forms of preventative exercise, you too can integrate a pre-habilitation programme into your weekly training regime and actually perform the very same exercises that the likes of Rooney, Ronaldo and Golden Balls himself do on a regular basis.

CORE STRENGTH AND STABILITY

Years ago, uttering the phrase 'core strength' would have ensured that you were greeted with quizzical looks from team-mates and physios alike. These days, the importance of a strong and balanced core is right at the top of the list of ways to prevent injuries to all structures from head to toe.

The core is a very complex area of human physiology and much misunderstood – even by many health professionals. Its structure and matrix of musculature has divided opinions among rehabilitation and conditioning experts. Some argue that players should concentrate far more on core conditioning to prevent injuries, while others believe that core conditioning is over-rated and that spending much time with it is unnecessary.

The general consensus, however, is that training the core muscles is a necessary part of pre-habilitation and does indeed play a vital role in stabilising the mid-section of the body in certain actions, such as those involved in subtly redirecting a header while keeping the body still. A stable core also means that peripheral muscles are not over-used and so are less likely to be injured.

It would be easy to write an entire book on the importance and the function of the core muscles in footballers and its significance in preventing injuries but for our purposes, I need only to give you an insight into some basic exercises to condition the core and to highlight the importance of how training with it can keep you off the physio's bench.

WHAT EXACTLY IS THE CORE?

Your core is essentially the collective name for the group of deep and superficial muscles in and around the mid-section of your body. To complicate matters, strictly speaking there are two different sections of the core – the inner unit and the outer unit.

THE INNER UNIT

The inner unit comprises four key muscles which help provide support for your back:

- Transversus abdominis
- Diaphragm
- Pelvic floor
- Multifidus (part of the inner core and an important

lower back muscle responsible for keeping the spine strong and preventing back injuries)

THE OUTER UNIT

● Rectus abdominis
● Internal obliques
● External obliques
● Latissimus dorsi
● Gluteus muscles

THE IMPORTANCE OF CONDITIONING THE INNER UNIT

Every player, from the Premiership to the Sunday league, should pay particular attention to the transversus abdominis. Of the four main inner unit muscles, this is the one to concentrate on toning and strengthening.

The transversus abdominis is a deep, corset-like muscle which acts in very much the same way as a corset. It helps to keep the stomach flat and more importantly for the footballer acts like a weights belt when you move, lunge, rotate or jump.

Or at least – it should.

For many people, not just footballers, this transversus abdominis muscle is sleepy and lies dormant. It is essential that this muscle is 'switched on' in footballers so that it can help support the fragile structures of the lower back. If it is unconditioned and inactive during activity it is unable to act as a support for the back and pelvis and can cause pelvic and spinal instability.

The consequence?

If you have been lazy in the gym or training paddock and

ignored the importance of working your transversus abdominis, effectively rendering it inactive, your back is far less well-protected whenever you make a sudden movement, leaving you exposed to an increased risk of injury. Additionally, a weak or inactive transversus abdominis can affect the stability of your pelvis and make it tilt forwards slightly.

No big deal you might think. But remember that your hamstring muscles are attached to your pelvis and this increased tilt can make them tauter and exposed to a greater risk of injury when you accelerate, something you do dozens of times every match.

These are just two examples of how a weak core can have a biomechanical effect on the rest of your body, increasing your chances of picking up an injury. Although it might sound a little far-fetched to suggest that training deep stomach muscles can prevent tearing a hamstring, it's a principle now accepted by all top clubs and a lot of work goes into ensuring every player has a fully-functional core to prevent injury.

The big question is how exactly do you train your deep core muscles?

There are a number of ways to do this but your best bet is to seek advice from a well qualified personal trainer who has a good understanding of core training. To give you something to get started on, try this basic exercise to wake up the transversus abdominis and get you started on a bit of core training.

● Suck in your stomach, so your belly button is drawn towards your spine

● Do not hold your breath – just keep breathing normally

You will know that you are doing this properly when you begin to feel a minor burning sensation in the deep stomach. This is a sign that the transversus abdominis has been engaged and is being worked. It's the same principle behind working your six-pack muscles while performing crunches. Initially, the transversus exercise is hard to do. Many people instinctively want to breathe in as they draw in the stomach, but with practice it gets easier. If you are still finding it difficult, try doing it on your hands and knees.

This exercise is the very basic form of deep core training and an essential one to get right before you move onto the more dynamic exercises – which are essential if you are to maximise your core's ability to protect your back during movement.

THE INNER UNIT, YOUR BRAIN AND YOUR BACK

There is another vital little gem of knowledge you need to know about conditioning your core. In preventing injuries it's important to train your deep core muscles while moving at the same time. If you don't, the core will be next to hopeless in preventing injury.

This was perfectly highlighted by a leading authority in sports conditioning who was invited to do an assessment on the fitness levels of a well-known sports team. He was assured by their head of fitness that the team's core strength was excellent. They had been working hard on it. Which was true, but not exactly in the way that guaranteed the best results.

When assessed, players did indeed demonstrate very good transversus abdominis function when lying down on the floor (the position in which most people perform their core exercises). But when they were made to integrate movement into their routine their core went to pieces and actually demonstrated significant weakness.

What had happened was a classic mistake that far too many people make. Despite the good intention they had for working those deep muscles, the players were doing their core exercises statically. They had conditioned their brains to switch on the deep stomach muscles when lying down on the floor, but it was not trained to engage the deep muscles when any movement was introduced. Hardly ideal when, for a footballer, the very reason you train your core is to work for you in running, jumping and changing direction.

So, when training your deep core muscles (and primarily your transversus abdominis), remember that in order to maximise protection for your back you ultimately need to teach the brain to engage them when moving – not just when lying down on a gym mat!

THE OUTER UNIT

The outer unit of the core is made up of a large number of muscles which move the trunk, such as your rectus abdominis muscles (the stomach muscles which give you a six-pack) your obliques situated on the side of the trunk and your major bum muscles.

They are like the inner unit in that it is essential to keep these muscles strong to help support your body when tearing around the pitch, changing direction and turning on a sixpence. If these muscles are weak you are not only failing to develop a decent support structure to protect your back but you are also making it far more difficult for yourself if you really want to be at the top of your game physically. By keeping the outer unit in good condition your body will be far more able to do what you want it to by rotating quickly, giving you increased stability and strength in the air, handing you a significant advantage over the opposition.

Be warned, though, when you undertake a regime of outer unit conditioning: it is possible to overdo it and cause injuries in other areas of the body. The classic example of this is an over-enthusiastic approach to sit-ups in the gym with the aim of strengthening the stomach and sculpting that much sought after six-pack which the chicks die for. The aesthetic appeal of a chiselled washboard stomach may very well help win the affections of a future WAG but for the sake of your overall structural health, keep down the number of abdominal crunches. This will help to prevent injury further up what's called the kinetic chain. This is a problem so many players fall victim to, so here is a brief explanation as to why you should try and resist going crazy on abdominal exercises.

When you exercise any muscle in the body, the contraction of the fibres make the muscle shorten – which is why you are encouraged to stretch before and after matches. Without stretching, muscles become shorter over time and eventually start pulling ever so slightly on the structures on which they are attached. Your stomach is no exception.

Real gym bunnies with an obsession for performing thousands of stomach crunches will gradually shorten the stomach muscles. Over a few weeks or even months, this shortening may not have a significant impact on your muscles but as they continue to shorten the stomach will start to flex your spine, putting it in a subtle forward-leaning position. This would barely be noticeable to the untrained eye but a physiotherapist would see it as an injury time-bomb waiting to go off.

This forward leaning posture makes the head protrude slightly and will also make the neck far more vulnerable to injury by affecting the balance of musculature in your trunk. To illustrate the point consider this example: let's say that you are a typical ab crunch-obsessed player who will do thousands of sit-ups every week and has done for years. Like most gym bunnies, you train your stomach in a number of ways, from crunches on floor to crunches in the ab cradle to support your neck.

You take to the football field with your rock hard abs, giving the girls a quick flash as you pass and getting ready to open a can of whoop-ass on the opposing team. Ten minutes in, when chasing back for the ball, you get unceremoniously checked from behind while going for a header, the full force of your opposite number's shoulder in your lower back.

This unexpected impact immediately engages your brain's natural instinct to protect the effect of the blow and sends signals to your body to counteract the force of the shoulder in your back by straightening up. Your brain switches on those well-trained ab muscles to flex forwards. And they are so well-conditioned and very used to flexing. Your body can do this easily – but what about your neck?

All those crunches in the gym performed with your head supported by your hands, or with that pad on the ab cradle, have caused a massive weakness in your neck-flexing muscles in relation to your bullet-bouncing, rock-hard abs. This violent check from behind your neck has left it vulnerable. It has far less strength and less ability to right itself after the impact.

This muscle imbalance can cause whiplash-style injuries and a host of other problems all over the body as a direct result of shortened and excessively strong abs in relation to other muscles. So if you thought the only way to prevent injuries was to do a few simple stretches before a game – think again.

WORK THAT BUTT

In direct contrast to over-training the stomach muscles and exposing yourself to the risk of injury, not paying enough attention to your ass is another common mistake made by all footballers. It can result in major problems, ranging from back pain to general instability in your running gait.

The nature of the game includes acceleration, direction changes and kicking of the ball and all repeated hundreds of times. You expose your body to some significant muscular imbalances which, over time, can result in injury.

Your butt muscles are essential for stabilising your body as it progresses through a running stride. If the group is weak in relation to other powerful muscles such as your thighs or hip flexors, the result can be a detrimental effect on the stability of your pelvis and may result in recurrent back pain and a variety of other problems.

DON'T IGNORE THE CORE
The effect that a weak core can have is massively significant and something you should always have in your mind when you are getting in shape for the season. If you really are serious about improving as a player I'd take your core training – inner and outer units – very seriously.

A leading strength and conditioning coach for a top Premiership club explained to me the essential role core training plays in preventing injuries. It is now a major feature of both pre-season and in-season preparations. Although, he added, a lot of players still find it hard to get their heads around and often find core exercises not nearly as exciting as other aspects of fitness. But word is getting around that it is now just as important as shuttle runs and weight training.

PROPRIOCEPTION AND INJURY PREVENTION
The use of proprioceptive training to help players in pre-habilitation and rehabilitation has been around decades – far longer than core training.

It's difficult to explain without going too scientific on you, but proprioception is basically the 'sixth sense' that your body and brain uses to know where you are in relation to the world. For example, you should be able to stand on an unstable surface in the gym, such as a Bosu platform, without falling off – albeit with some difficulty. You might be wobbling about all over the place but due to the feedback your brain gets from all your senses, you instinctively know how to very quickly balance yourself to stabilise.

This process of continually shifting balancing is not under your conscious control. Your brain does all the work without active thought, rapidly contracting one muscle and relaxing another, to keep you balanced on the uneven surface.

When you get injured, the information that is sent to the brain will also not be as good as that of a healthy subject. The brain would lose proprioception in an injured ankle very quickly, for example, and that will affect the ability to balance. You'll notice that even when the pain and swelling has gone, standing on that part of your body for any length of time is virtually impossible.

Of course, the big question is: what impact and benefit does proprioception training have on a footballer? If the game is played on a level surface then what is the point in training the brain to stand on a wobbly platform?

Proprioception is predominantly neurological: i.e., it requires that the brain reacts instinctively to a sensation of imbalance and makes the body move to a more stable position, ultimately to prevent injury. And when you do happen to be injured, the specific training helps you to recover. This is where the use of proprioception training is hugely beneficial to the footballer, particularly one coming back from an ankle or knee injury.

In times of instability on the pitch, such as when you land on one leg after jumping up to head the ball, poor proprioception means you will be unable to react quickly to engage the lower leg muscles and prevent the ankle from rolling over. By working in the gym on proprioception exercises, you can really condition the brain and lower leg muscles to better tolerate those times of instability.

Studies carried out on the benefits of proprioception training for the prevention of ankle injuries have shown clear evidence that those players who perform it regularly have a far lesser risk of picking up injuries than those who don't.

HOW DOES IT WORK?

The process of proprioception training, thankfully, is far easier than working out what the word actually means.

The best way to do it is simply to stand on an unstable surface – such as a wobble board or stability disc at the gym. This might be hard to do at first but the more time you spend on it the more your brain will be trained to know how to regain stability.

Over time you will start to find the basics easy so you can improve your proprioception by:

- Performing arm exercises such as dumbbell curls or lateral raises to make you more unstable on the disc
- Perform the same exercises with one arm at a time to cause further imbalance, taxing the brain and balancing muscles a little more
- Stand on the wobble platform on one leg
- Perform a series of arm exercises on the unstable surface while standing on one leg.

Injured or not, all players can benefit from regular proprioception training. It's a fun way to work out and if it's performed regularly you will give yourself every chance of preventing ankle and knee injuries.

FINAL WORD ON PRE-HABILITATION

Although you don't have the luxury of free, 24-hour access to exercise and rehabilitation specialists, you should now have a far better idea on how to go about protecting yourself from injury. You may not have the money to spare for a great deal of specialist advice, but if you can, I'd strongly recommend at least a consultation or two with a highly qualified trainer or injury specialist. They will be able to do a few quick tests to spot potential muscle imbalances which could result in an injury at any time.

Of course, you can do all the 'prehab' you like, give yourself a stronger core than Hercules and condition your proprioception to the max, but football remains a contact sport. Cop a double footed tackle on your knee and you could be nursing torn ligaments or tendons for weeks.

Injuries like these are unavoidable. But there are a number of steps you can take to reduce your time wallowing in self-pity and get yourself back on the pitch.

ANATOMY OF A FOOTBALLER

You might currently be injured and reading this chapter for advice on playing again or simply looking for a few tips on how to avoid contracting your next injury. Either way, it helps if you develop an understanding of the most popular injuries and learn the names and locations of the major muscles prone to injury.

You've probably discovered that as soon as you're injured your mates come out with wonderful words of advice. These 'informed' gems down the local pub may include 'Rub this gel on it', 'Try this bandage' and the ever popular: 'Get the wife to rub it better, ha, ha, ha.' The big question is – do they actually know what they are talking about?

Granted a massage from your better half, if you can get it, will go a long way towards getting you on the road to recovery. But for the vast majority who fail in that quest, the following section will pass on the very advice that top Premiership physios give for treating an injury – without the use of high-tech equipment.

The problem with listening to friends is that they probably get their knowledge from a magazine article or another friend and the quality – and accuracy – is thus very questionable. Follow the advice in this section of the book and you will have peace of mind. The protocols described are pretty much identical to that followed by a leading Premiership physio.

You'll be out playing one hell of a lot sooner, especially if you manage to bag a massage from your better half as well!

THE LEG MUSCLES – A CLOSER LOOK
First things first.

Before you can even begin to go about treating an injury by yourself, it is important that you know a little bit of anatomy. By learning the whereabouts of certain leg muscles and ligaments, you'll be far better placed to what exactly is injured and be far better placed to treat it effectively.

The majority of people, even those who have little interest in exercise, have a certain amount of knowledge about leg muscles. Most people have heard of the quads, or quadriceps, and the hamstrings but few are aware that the bigger picture is a little more complex.

The table below outlines some of the commonly-known leg muscle groups on the left and a more detailed look at the muscles and structures that make up that group on the right.

Muscle group	Divisions
Quadriceps	vastus medialis
	vastus intermedialis
	vastus lateralis
	rectus femoris
Hamstrings	bicep femoris
	semimembranosus
	semitendonosis
Calf muscles	gastrocnemius
	soleus
Adductors	magnus
	brevis
	longus
	gracilis
Gluteals	maximus
	minimus
	medius

Other individual muscles, tendons and ligaments which are prone to injury include:

- Achilles tendon
- Illio tibial band (ITB)
- Talo-fibular ligament (ankle)
- Calcaneofibular ligament (ankle)
- Hernia

MUSCLE AND LIGAMENT INJURIES

Although recent England players such as Wayne Rooney and David Beckham have popularised metatarsal injuries with the help of highly excited tabloid articles featuring pictures of their feet for us to kiss better in the run up to World Cup matches, by far the most common types of injuries are muscle tears and ligament sprains. It is these I am going to focus on and help you to cure fast.

If I had to give a top five of the most common injuries in football, they would be:

- Hamstring strain
- Adductor strain
- Ankle sprain
- Medial collateral ligament sprain
- Anterior cruciate ligament sprain

The good news is that due to the 'popularity' of such injuries there is quite a range of treatments for you to buy. However, do not fall for the belief that you can make the injury heal quicker than nature intended simply by spending £100 on a bandage here and £50 on a rub-on gel there. Certain products help, but first you need to assess the degree of damage you have suffered. Only then will you be in a position to pick and choose pills and potions to speed things along.

Whether you tear a muscle or a ligament the treatment in the early stages is very similar, but you must learn the subtle differences between the two structures.

SERIOUS TEAR – OR BIG GIRL'S BLOUSE?

The vast majority of injuries occur during a match when muscle or ligament tears are likely to be caused by a dodgy tackle or sudden burst of acceleration.

As all football fans will know, watching Premiership games on the TV, it is often impossible to tell the severity of an injury when a player goes down clutching his injured limb – not least because of the theatrics which go on in and around the box. In your case you'll know when something has torn as the pain can be excruciating and the notion of playing on will simply not be an option.

When you injure your knee, ankle or hamstring the first thing you need to do, apart from apply ice, is to assess the severity of the tear.

The degree of damage is generally classed as a grade of tear in the following way:

GRADE 1

A small number of muscle or ligament fibres are torn, causing minor discomfort. In cases of a muscle tear, bleeding is small and normal function is possible and you should be able to walk around – albeit tentatively.

GRADE 2

A large number of fibres are torn causing significant pain and an inability to walk properly. There is significant bleeding within the area of the injury and palpation is painful. Muscle and/or joint function is impaired and the level of discomfort is significant enough for you not to be branded as a big girl's blouse when you whinge about the pain you are in.

GRADE 3

A severe tear in which the majority of the muscle or ligament fibres have ruptured. There is a large degree of bleeding or swelling which can spread over a large area. Muscle or joint movement is impaired and the pain is excruciating – especially to touch.

GRADE 4

A complete muscle or ligament rupture is highly uncommon but if it happens, you can probably wave your season goodbye –whether you play in the Premiership or a Sunday League team. The muscle or ligament is completely torn away from the bone and a 'snapping' sound can sometimes be heard. If you do completely rupture a muscle you will certainly know about it.

INITIAL INJURY MANAGEMENT

Whether it is a ligament or muscle which suddenly tears during a game, it is essential that you get yourself off the pitch and treated.

Trying to man up and keep playing on a grade 1 ankle, hamstring or knee injury may be the initial reaction of the hardcore player but – for the good of your team and the injury itself – get yourself off the field and the injury treated. Once a muscle or ligament has torn, playing on it is only going to make it worse. Adrenaline can help you through the pain, but the longer you play the more likely you are to increase the grade of your injury – extending your time out of the game by a further 4-6 weeks.

ICE, ICE BABY

Although the majority of players now know that ice is the best treatment for injuries, for years they believed that a hot water bottle or heat lamp was the best medicine for a hamstring or ankle injury. While heat can be applied in the more chronic stages of injury, ice has to become your best friend for at least the initial two days following an injury – and probably longer. Although the feeling might not be as comforting as the feel of a nice hot water bottle, if you want to get back playing you have to become obsessed with icing your injury.

Why?

It's all down to how the capillaries respond to cold after the fibres have been torn.

When you strain, pull or tear a muscle or ligament, bruising breaks out. It is the visible results of the broken blood vessels. The severity and size of the bruise will vary depending on the size of the trauma and severity of the injury, but even in minor cases when a bruise may not even be visible, a number of blood vessels will still be bleeding within the muscle.

It is when these blood vessels are still bleeding that you need to avoid applying anything hot to the area. The application of heat encourages the broken blood vessels to dilate, allowing even more blood to flow to the area. This not only delays the healing process but also makes the bruise spread. It's the equivalent of turning the taps on to stop a bath from over-flowing.

As unpleasant as it might feel, the best thing you can do to reduce the flow of blood from the broken blood vessels is to apply ice in any way you can. A packet of frozen peas, an ice bucket or a high-tech ice boot – such as that used by Premiership players – it doesn't matter how you do it, just get ice on that injury and keep using at it until the swelling has gone down.

If you fancy taking this procedure of blood-vessel constriction a little further, try relaxing in a soothing, toe-curling ice bath after picking up an injury or after a game. Though fantastic for your muscles and something every team should adopt to help with muscle repair and recovery, it's not so great for the male ego when it comes to the shrinkage issue associated with cold water and men's bits.

However, believe it or not, there is a right way and a wrong way to ice an injury. Opinion differs, but it is generally thought that to work most effectively ice should not be placed on the injury for longer than 20 minutes, as the body will adapt to the cool environment. You should also take a break before reapplying. Experts are in some disagreement about the amount of time to leave between sessions, but anywhere between 20 minutes and an hour is generally regarded to be the norm.

EARLY TREATMENT FOR MUSCLE AND LIGAMENT TEARS

The procedures for treating the early stages of a muscle or ligament tear are very similar. The only notable difference is that with ligament injuries due to their avascular nature (they have no blood supply) the use of heat in the latter stages of treatment may need to be prolonged. Ligaments are incredibly stubborn to treat due to this lack of blood, so you just have to be that much more patient.

HAMSTRING AND ADDUCTORS

Hamstring tears accounted for a whopping 40 per cent of total Premiership injuries in the 2006/2007 season and there is no reason why that trend will not continue for the foreseeable future.

In footballers, the hamstrings are under enormous strain during periods of acceleration. If a biomechanical problem causes them to be constantly taut or if you have failed to do a proper warm-up, the hamstrings may even rip. You could then be sidelined for weeks.

As for the adductors, commonly referred to as the groin, many players injure them with annoying regularity over the course of their career. Like the hamstrings, the adductors are put under enormous strain when you sprint and if you have neglected to stretch them or warm up properly prior to a match, you are asking for trouble.

You can illustrate the difference in the adductor muscle recruitment when you jog and sprint by doing an exercise next time you are on hols and running on the beach. Jog up one way in wet sand and take a note of the foot imprints you leave. You'll notice that there are two lines of prints – you can clearly see the prints of your feet on the left and on the right of your running line. Now do a sprint back alongside your prints and you'll notice that your feet will leave just one line of prints. The faster you run the more narrow your running line gets – courtesy of the recruitment of your adductor muscles.

You spend a considerable amount of time sprinting and accelerating and your adductors are workhorses. They need to be looked after if you are to stay off the physio's bench and out on the pitch playing.

ANKLE AND KNEE SPRAINS

Along with hamstring injuries, ankle sprains are incredibly common amongst players and account for around 25 per cent of all footballing injuries. They are one of those injuries which can happen without anyone near you and the healing process can be incredibly frustrating due to the lack of blood supply to the ligaments.

Knee injuries to both the ligament on the inside of the knee (medial collateral ligament) and outside of the knee (lateral collateral ligament) are usually as a result of a side-on tackle and, if severe, can lead to further complication within the knee joint. These may affect the cartilage and have the potential to cause long-term damage.

Whereas good warm-ups, correct stretching and core conditioning can help prevent muscle tears, many ligament injuries are unavoidable. It's just the price you pay for playing an intense, multi-directional sport. Highly specific strength training and proprioception exercises can certainly help, but if the opposing central defender targets your knee or ankle with both feet and a smile on his face, there is not a lot you can do.

INJURIES: THE FIRST 48 HOURS

The sensation of a muscle or ligament tear depends very much on the severity.

The sound of a grade 4 total hamstring rupture has been likened to that of a gun being fired – but your luck would have to be really poor if that were to happen to you during play. Total ruptures during a match are rarer than rocking horse poop, so if you do get one I'd go and buy a lottery ticket to even out your fortunes. Most of the time you will suffer either a grade 1 or grade 2 tear but don't let the rating fool you – you'll certainly know about it.

The tear is likely to occur during a sudden burst of acceleration and your immediate reaction will be to grab hold of the back of the injured leg and hobble around. I've told you before – get your butt off the pitch as soon as you can and get the ice on the injury. You don't see Premiership players hobbling around the pitch for long after picking up a hamstring injury so why should you be any different? Once it has snapped it has snapped. It's not going to get any better if you hop around with a pained expression like Quasimodo!

Once off the pitch, keep the affected area elevated and iced and try to resist the temptation to jump up and down if/when your side scores.

After the game has finished and you've showered (keeping heat off the injured area), repaired to the bar (with ice on the injury) and are wallowing in self pity, take some time to get your head around the fact that the next 48 hours will be crucial to recovering from injury.

The procedure is the same as it was in the first 48 minutes. Ice, ice and more ice – alongside procedures that top physios use on Premiership players.

The acronym RICE comes into play for at least two days after the injury – and sometimes up to three or four days – to ensure the knitting of muscle fibres can begin as soon as possible. RICE has been used for years by footballers, but in recent times the top physios have adapted the acronym to PRICE –MM and there is no reason why you too can't use the new injury protocol to treat your war wounds. So – what do those letters mean?

PROTECTION
It is essential to keep the site of injury safe from potential further damage. Protecting it from being knocked or bumped is a key precaution to reduce the risk of further damage.

REST
Avoid training the injured area for – at the very least – 48-72 hours to allow the swelling to go down.

ICE

Apply an ice pack or a bag of frozen peas to the injured muscle or joint. This helps to narrow the capillaries and stop the muscle from bleeding.

COMPRESSION

Use a bandage or piece of tight clothing to compress the muscle. This helps to reduce swelling and bleeding.

ELEVATION

Elevate the injured muscle above your heart in order to reduce blood flow to the bleeding muscle.

MM

Medication and modalities are the final part of the acronym and arguably the most important. Anti-inflammatories can speed up recovery time, although they should not be relied upon and care must be taken to follow the correct dosage.

Following the PRICE part of the protocol is essential whoever you are and is an invaluable part of getting the healing process underway. However, it is only in the Premiership where the MM of treatment can truly be maximised.

With easy access to doctors and highly-qualified physiotherapists, the boys of the Premiership can be assessed and given the correct types and dosages of NSAIDs (Non-Steroidal Anti-Inflammatory Drugs). Their injuries are also treated with high-tech electrical stimulation machines. Without access to this level of expertise it is potentially dangerous to self-administer NSAIDs, despite the fact that they can be purchased over the counter.

Although dedication to your sport and team may encourage you to get back out there as soon as possible, taking excessive doses of NSAIDs is not only pointless but potentially dangerous. What many people do not know is that one of the side-effects of common anti-inflammatory drugs is that they can literally burn holes in your stomach, giving you internal bleeding and ulcers when not used properly. The pros have the luxury of being monitored and given exactly the correct amount of medication to prevent side effects and to maximise their healing – you don't. So either seek proper medical advice or at least think twice about popping anti-inflammatories as if they were Smarties – stick to the ice.

BEYOND 48 HOURS

After 48 hours treatment can generally move onto the next phase – heat. By the time 48 hours are up, the swelling and bleeding in your hamstring/adductor or ankle/knee should have reduced – but this won't be true in every case. If the injury is quite severe or you have been a little lax with your PRICE, there is every chance that you will have to leave it another 48 hours.

So how do you know when to move on from only using the ice pack and onto heat?

The clue is really in the swelling. Once the swelling has stopped or started to go down then you are ready to reduce the amount of time you ice the area and go on to applying heat –as long as you then reapply the ice pack. However, if you are unsure, it is best to stick with ice for another 24 hours.

In this crucial stage of healing, the general advice is to

follow a minute of heat on the injured area with three minutes of cold. The process can be repeated up to five times. Always end with a five-minute cold compress.

The use of heat is an invaluable modality to encourage blood flow. This rush of blood brings with it vital nutrients and enzymes which help the muscle fibres repair themselves and knit together. It is especially important for ligaments, which do not have their own blood supply and will take an age to heal. You need to do all you can to attract blood to the area.

AFTER THE FIRST WEEK

A week or so after the initial injury, provided you have followed protocol, the swelling should have gone down significantly (preferably altogether) and you are ready to increase your use of heat on the area.

In this third stage of injury treatment, you should be looking to treat the area with two minutes of ice followed by two minutes of heat. Repeat this up to five times and always conclude with a five-minute cold compress.

The more you treat the area with ice and heat the better. This continuous contracting and dilating of the blood vessels helps to stimulate the delivery of huge amounts of blood to the area. It gives the injury nutrients and enzymes to stitch up the muscle or ligament fibres and get them back to working order again.

As long as swelling does not return, you can continue to increase the number of times you apply heat to the area – *but not for longer than ten minutes*. Going over ten minutes can bring on swelling and potentially set you back a stage in the healing process.

By now you should start to feel a lot better but it is important to continue with heat treatment for a number of days to ensure the fibres heal properly. Remember, ligaments take far longer to heal than muscles so expect to keep treating the area of up to two weeks and beyond.

INTRODUCING EXERCISE

Knowing what sort of exercise to do when injured is often very tricky.

In the very early stages, depending on the severity of the trauma, it is best to elevate the injury to keep the swelling under control. However, in the second and third stages of treatment top physios suggest very gentle exercise and stretching to the muscles to help prevent the formation of scar tissue. It is best to do these during your icing treatments and, in the case of ankle sprains, to roll the foot in different directions to keep it mobile and the scar tissue to a minimum.

Even once you are able to walk or gently run, be cautious and build up the exercise intensity gradually over a series of days. Leg exercises help to strengthen torn hamstring and adductor muscles but these should be done incredibly gently and preferably under the guidance of a trained physiotherapist.

Although a series of static leg exercises (keeping the injured muscle under contraction for ten seconds or so) can be helpful in the rehabilitation stage, moving on to a series of dynamic muscle exercises can be the best way to complete the rehabilitation of the injured area. It is nevertheless advisable to seek professional help to ensure there are no complications with your particular injury.

Although the financial implications might put you off, often a single trip to a specialist can be invaluable. They will advise you on the best form of treatment and rehabilitation to get you back on the pitch as soon as possible. If you have meticulously followed the advice in the PRICE-MM protocol you will have already saved yourself a bundle of cash, so make sure the final stages of your injury are treated correctly. Physiotherapists or sports therapists can tell you how to do the stretching and strengthening exercises which are specific to your injury. They will be able to give you advice on how to look after your injury and they will reiterate the importance of good rehabilitation.

Fibres in the hamstrings, adductor, ankle and knee will be weakened after an injury, even when they've knitted back together. You are likely to face the same problem again unless you're extremely conscientious with your rehab. It's essential to look after the muscle by doing regular specific rehab exercises even when it has repaired.

FINDING A THERAPIST

If an injury or niggle becomes a chronic problem, consulting a professional is the most logical step to take. The dilemma faced by many players, however, is who to go to for treatment.

Physiotherapists, chiropractors, sports therapists and massage therapists are just a few of the specialists who commonly help to treat injuries. Personal recommendation is without doubt the best form of referral. If a friend has been successfully treated for an injury by a certain therapist, it is likely that the same practitioner will be able to help you.

Make sure that whoever treats your injury has the correct qualifications and insist on knowing what they believe the exact nature of your injury is and how long they think it will take to heal. If your injury is similar to any of the conditions mentioned, it is always a good idea to inform the therapist what you think it may be so that they realise you have a degree of knowledge.

Parting with money for receiving treatment that is not working not only hits you in the wallet but is a waste of potential training time. If you feel your injury is not improving as quickly as you would expect, let your feelings be known to the therapist and if necessary seek a second opinion.

Different practitioners have areas of specialisation:

PHYSIOTHERAPISTS

They treat soft tissue injuries, such as ligament, muscle and tendon tears. They use ultrasound, massage, stretching and manipulation.

CHIROPRACTORS

Through spinal manipulation, with an emphasis on correct spinal and pelvic alignment, they help correct some biomechanical injuries. They manipulate the spine to correct vertebral and pelvic misalignments.

MASSAGE THERAPIST

A massage therapist will do deep tissue massage to help elongate muscle fibres and disperse knotted muscles. They